# My Telephone On-Call Experience

## Pediatric Advice and Triage

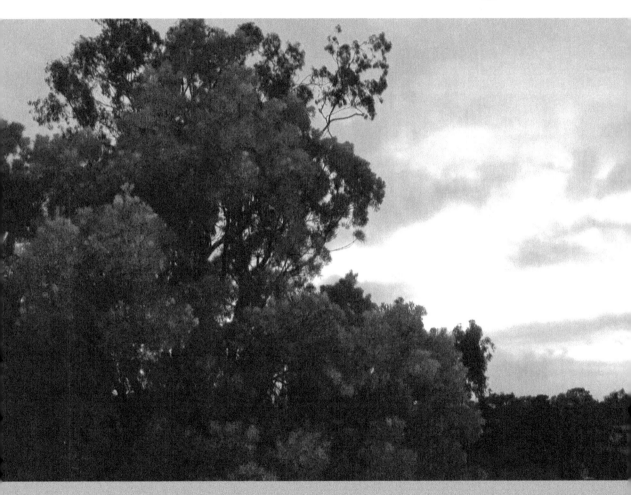

# Shahnaz Zomorrodian Erfani, M.D., FAAP

### Seamae Eghtedari Erfani, MD, Editor

Outskirts Press, Inc.
http://www.outskirtspress.com

ISBN: 978-1-4787-9381-6

Editor: Seamae Eghtedari Erfani, MD

Outskirts Press and the "OP" logo are trademarks belonging to Outskirts Press, Inc.

PRINTED IN THE UNITED STATES OF AMERICA

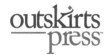

# TABLE OF CONTENTS

Introduction . . . . . . . . . . . . . . . . . . . . . . . . . .i

Preface . . . . . . . . . . . . . . . . . . . . . . . . . . . .iii

Chapter One . . . . . . . . . . . . . . . . . . . . . . . 1
Cases #1-50

Chapter Two . . . . . . . . . . . . . . . . . . . . . . .21
Cases #51-100

Chapter Three . . . . . . . . . . . . . . . . . . . . . .41
Cases #51-100

Chapter Four . . . . . . . . . . . . . . . . . . . . . . .62
Cases #151-200

Chapter Five . . . . . . . . . . . . . . . . . . . . . . .85
Cases #201-250

Chapter Six . . . . . . . . . . . . . . . . . . . . . . . 107
Cases #251-300

Chapter Seven . . . . . . . . . . . . . . . . . . . . . 129
Cases #301-350

Chapter Eight . . . . . . . . . . . . . . . . . . . . . . 150
Cases #351-400

Chapter Nine . . . . . . . . . . . . . . . . . . . . . . 171
Cases #401-450

Chapter Ten . . . . . . . . . . . . . . . . . . . . . . . 192
Cases #451-500

Chapter Eleven . . . . . . . . . . . . . . . . . . . . 212
Cases #501-550

Chapter Twelve . . . . . . . . . . . . . . . . . . . . 233
Case #551-600

Chapter Thirteen . . . . . . . . . . . . . . . . . . . 255
Case #601-635

The Chief Complaints Alphabetically . . . . . . . . . . 272

About the Author . . . . . . . . . . . . . . . . . . . 290

About the Editor . . . . . . . . . . . . . . . . . . . 291

Acknowledgements . . . . . . . . . . . . . . . . . . . 292

# Introduction

By Dr. Seamae Erfani

When growing up as a daughter of a pediatrician, I distinctly remember my mother's pager going off. There were many weekends that my mother would be "on call" from home for 24 hours at a time, taking calls from mostly mothers and fathers about their children's symptoms and ailments. Without fail my mother would take out her notebook, call them back immediately, listen while taking notes, and answer all their questions. She would have them repeat the instructions back to her, and end with "Do you have any other questions or concerns you would like me to address?"

I did not mind sharing my mother with the thousands of children who she would help throughout the years. In fact, I was as proud of her then as I am now, because of her dedication to Pediatrics and its advancement. The joy that helping families brought to her was infectious. It was no surprise then, when I decided to follow in her small but mighty footsteps.

And when I became a pediatrician myself many years later, my pager now replaced by iPhones, I saw that having access to a trusted pediatrician's advice via telephone is still something parents seek out.

Parents, grandparents and caregivers continue to want answers to their questions regarding child rearing, reassurance, and guidance when their children are ill.
With this in mind, my mother decided she would like to write about the 30 years of experience she had as a practicing pediatrician in New York (the Bronx). The advice she rendered to these families, first over the rotary phone and later over a cordless

phone, is still as relevant today as it was 30 years ago, despite the constantly changing nature of medicine.

I am extremely proud of my mother now, as I was then, for her dedication to this project. It is both an honor and privilege that she has asked me to edit her manuscript, which follows in the pages ahead.

# PREFACE

Protecting and advancing the well-being of children and young adults is a key responsibility of pediatricians. Children and adolescents are a vulnerable group in society due to their lacking the ability to care for themselves and because as minors, they are often not given a voice. About one third of the world's population consists of children, adolescents, and young adults.

Likewise, in the United States, it was estimated that in 2015, children under five years of age made up 6.6% of the total population, children between five to thirteen 11.4%, adolescents fourteen to seventeen years of age 5.2%, and those eighteen to twenty-four made up 9.6% of the total population. It is imperative to help keep children and young adults in good health, physically, mentally, and emotionally to produce healthy, happy, and productive adults.

There are many facets to the Pediatrics specialty. The pediatrician through counseling and guidance, recommendations on safety, nutrition, immunizations, and healthy habits like hygiene and exercise can have a large impact on the health of children and families. Pediatricians have a great deal of ground to cover over the years, and so many have sustained positive impacts on the well-being of children and adolescents.

In this collection of my telephone on-call notes, I will focus my attention on the specific problems that mothers and caregivers were facing during the off-hours of the pediatric clinics and offices and problem solving by the caring pediatrician. It is important to realize which cases must be seen earlier at the hospital emergency department (ED). Please keep in mind that during the time of these calls, urgent care facilities were not as common as they are now.

The on-call physician should make sound decisions to prevent unnecessary trips to the ED at night and avoid an extra burden to the hospital, curtail healthcare expenses, as well as to decrease the stressors of the family with wait times and potential exposure to infectious diseases. At the same time, and of paramount importance, the physician must strive to provide the best of care for the patient.

In the chapters ahead, I provide the contents of the notes and the advice given while serving as an on-call pediatrician. The calls have been arranged by the season and the time of the calls. I should mention that the calls are not sequential but take place over several years. I have left out any identifying factors.

Please note the timing of the calls because a call in the early morning may be advised to get checked on the same day in clinic only because that would be easy and feasible, while someone with the same ailment calling in the evening, may, according to the severity of the case, be advised to be seen on next day and not the same night at the ED to prevent over-crowding the emergency department.

The cases are some of my notes that I kept during a few of my years of night calls. I am optimistic that writing and presenting these cases to others including my own daughter who is a pediatrician and a mother, will be educational and beneficial.

Certain conditions do have seasonal variability. Some ailments may have the same chief complaints but the medical decision- making would differ based on the age of the child.

In this book, I have referred to the "neonate" as the infant from birth to age four to six weeks. The "infant" will refer to children between one month and 12-14 month of age. I will refer to "toddlers" as children aged between 14 months to 3 years. Cases involving children aged 4-12 years will be referred to as those of the school-aged child or simply "child." And cases involving children aged 13-21 years will be referred to as those of "adolescents."
I want to thank all the families that allowed me to help care for their children in the years I served them.

I also thank my daughter and the editor of this book, Dr. Seamae Eghtedari Erfani, she herself a dedicated mother and pediatrician, for her nice introduction and time.

I do not intend for the words in this book to be used to treat one's child or to be used in the place of taking the child to be checked or seeking advice from a physician;

rather just as a means of sharing my experiences. I do hope that mothers and fathers, pediatricians, and family practitioners, telephone triage receptionists, and nurses will all gain something from the reading of my notes and that it helps them in some way.

Shahnaz Zomorrodian Erfani, M.D., FAAP

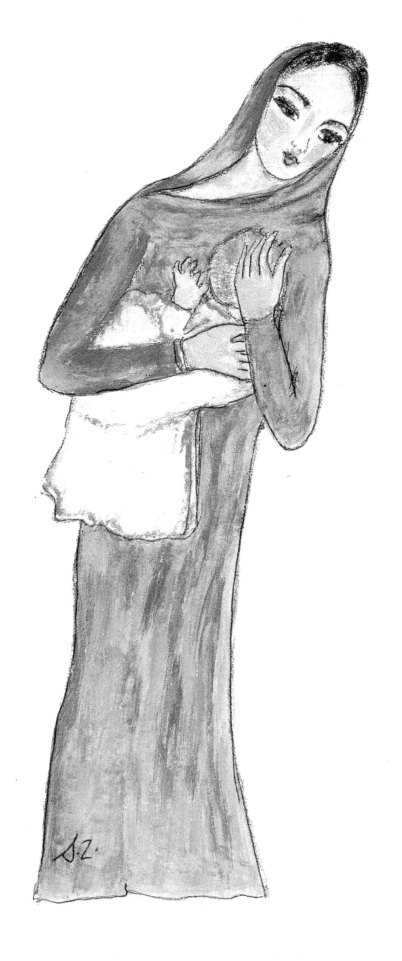

# CHAPTER ONE

## CASE #1

MID-SUMMER EVENING                                              TIME: 7:39PM

A one-year-old male infant

Chief complaint (CC): Head injury/fall
The child fell from the arms of his 10-year-old cousin about one and a half hours ago, hitting his head on the ground. His father denies any loss of consciousness and he had no vomiting. The father states that the child's head hit the concrete with a sound and that he now has some swelling, an ice pack has been applied.
Disposition: The father is advised to take the infant to the hospital to be checked. Because of his having fallen on concrete, as well as the height of the fall, a sound having been heard by the father, the age of the child, and the presence of a possible hematoma, it is important to have the child checked the same night.

## CASE #2

MID-SUMMER EVENING                                              TIME: 8:32PM

A ten-month-old female infant

CC: Crying & holding her ears
The mother states that the infant has had a temperature 100.9°F (38.2°C) for the last two or three days. She had called and spoken to a physician and was advised to observe the infant. The infant is currently afebrile (without fever) and has had no vomiting but has been cranky and is holding her ears.

1

Disposition: The mother is advised that if the infant has no fever she can take the child to be examined tomorrow at clinic given that there has been ear pulling.

## Case #3

A three-year-old female

CC: Fever & vomiting
The child's mother is concerned that the toddler has been sick off-and-on for the past two months. She received a course of antibiotic (Biaxin) about two weeks ago because of a throat infection. Today, she has had a fever and has vomited. She also has several mosquito bites on her body.
Disposition: The mother is advised to offer the child an antipyretic (fever reducer) like Children's Tylenol and fluid like juice, soup, ginger ale and to observe the child. If she is unable to tolerate fluid or is not urinating at least every 6-8 hours, then the child can be seen at the hospital tonight. Otherwise, the child may be checked in the morning in clinic, given the symptom duration.

## Case #4

Mid-winter morning                                                    Time: 7:23AM

A six-month-old female infant

CC: Fever
The infant had a slight fever last night and has been sneezing.
This morning, she has temperature 103.0°F (39.4°C).
Disposition: The mother is advised to give the infant a dose of Tylenol and to take her to the walk-in clinic to be checked today, given the young age and the fever ≥102.2°F (39.0°C).

## Case #5

Mid-winter midnight                                                    Time: 12:02AM

A four-year-old female child (calling from out of state)

CC: Fever
The child's father states that the child has a temperature of 102.0°F (38.8°C) and

that Tylenol and cold syrup has been given to her. She has had no vomiting. The father is advised to avoid giving mixed cold medicine with Tylenol. In fact, 1t is not advisable for children 6 years old and under to take over-the-counter (OTC) cough and cold medications. He is advised to give the child fluid and a simple antipyretic like ibuprofen (Children's Motrin) or acetaminophen (Children's Tylenol) for the fever. Disposition: The child may be checked in the morning by a physician if she is worsening or not improving (in that state, as the child is out of state).

## CASE #6

MID-WINTER LATE AT NIGHT                                          TIME: 11:40PM

A three-month-old female infant

CC: Congestion & possible fever
The mother states that the infant's temperature was taken orally today and is 99.9°F (37.7°C). A pacifier thermometer has been used. She has been cranky and is spitting up the formula. She has a congested nose. The problems just started today.
Disposition: The mother is advised to use a humidifier and Normal Saline nose drops and observe. The nasal passages will be cleared with the use of the nose drops allowing the infant to breathe from her nose in lieu of her mouth, and her crankiness will be alleviated. A true fever is when the temperature is ≥100.4°F (38.0°C), and for this age, a rectal temperature is more accurate.
If the infant were to have a true fever and vomiting, or if she is very cranky, then she should be seen at the ED tonight. Otherwise, if there is no true fever and the oral intake and fussiness improve with the use of the Nasal Saline, then the child may be seen tomorrow.

## CASE #7

MID-WINTER NIGHT                                                   TIME: 9:24PM

A three-year-old female child

 CC: Fever & cough
The child has a fever, runny nose and a cough that started today. She has no vomiting. Her temperature is 102.0°F (38.8°C).
Disposition: Her mother is advised to give her a teaspoon of ibuprofen (Children's Motrin) and offer her fluid.
The toddler may be checked tomorrow morning.

## CASE #8

MID-WINTER NIGHT                                    TIME: 10:47PM

A two-year-old female child

CC: Rash with swelling of the ears & right ankle
The child has swelling of her ears and right ankle. She was seen by a physician today and is on oral Benadryl, but it appears that she is not responding and the rash is getting worse. The child is also an asthmatic and has some cough.
Disposition: Her mother is advised to start her asthma medicine (albuterol) and observe. However, if the condition is not getting better, she should be seen at the ED.


## CASE #9

MID-WINTER EVENING                                  TIME: 6:00PM

A two-year-old female child

CC: Eye discharge
The child has some eye discharge that started today, she has no fever.
Disposition: Her mother is advised to clean the eyes with sterile water and to observe. If the condition persists, then the toddler is to be examined tomorrow. If there is eyelash mattering (lashes stuck shut with discharge), this is suggestive of pink eye. However, given the young age of the child, it is better for the child to be seen so that the ears may be examined, especially if there are concomitant cold symptoms or if the discharge persists.


## CASE #10

MID-WINTER NIGHT                                    TIME: 8:26PM

A five-year-old female child

CC: Cold & history of bronchial asthma
Her mother states that the child has had a cold for two days and she has an underlying history of bronchial asthma. There is no respiratory distress (no fast breathing, no difficulty breathing, no use of abdominal muscles, or muscles around the ribs to breathe).
Disposition: The mother is advised to help the child use her asthma medication (albuterol) via the nebulizer as instructed, and to use Normal Saline nose drops in her nostrils. She should encourage her to drink fluid and observe. The mother is to take

the child in to be checked tomorrow if required, if the child does not develop signs of distress overnight which would require immediate care.

## CASE #11
MID-WINTER  TIME: 5:55PM

An eleven-month-old female infant

CC: Fever
The mother states that the infant has a fever. She had a temperature of 101.0°F (38.3°C) last night and her mother called the physician. She was given advice last night and the infant has been under observation. Tonight, she has developed a higher temperature of 102.0°F (38.8°C), and she is refusing to drink.
Disposition: Her mother is advised to give her acetaminophen (Tylenol) and fluid. If the temperature comes down and the infant takes the fluid well, then the infant may be checked tomorrow morning. If there is no response to the medication, or if she continues to refuse to drink, and does not urinate every 6 hours, then she should be checked at the ED tonight.

## CASE #12
MID-WINTER  TIME: 5:10PM

An eight-year-old female child

CC: Vomiting & headache
The mother states that the child had vomited today and has been complaining of a headache. The mother denies that the child has had any fever or diarrhea. She has a history of headache in the past.
Disposition: The mother is advised to give her ibuprofen (Children's Motrin 100mg/5mL) two teaspoons every 6-8 hours for headache, to offer her clear fluid like Pedialyte, and to observe. If the condition persists and is worsening, she may be seen at an ED tonight, otherwise it is best to have her checked tomorrow morning.

## CASE #13
MID-WINTER  TIME: 7:35AM

An eight-year-old male child

CHAPTER ONE                                                                 5

CC: Fever & an asthma attack

The mother states that the child has a fever and an asthma attack.

Disposition: The mother is advised to start giving him his asthma medication (albuterol) and acetaminophen (Children's Tylenol 160mg/5mL) every 4-6 hours for the fever. If the child is responding well and appears to be getting better, then they may continue the asthma medications and have him checked today at the walk-in clinic. If the child is in distress he may be taken to the ED.

## CASE #14

EARLY SPRING                                                      TIME: 7:40AM

A three-year-old male child

CC: Fever & an asthma attack

The mother states that the child has a fever and an asthma attack.

Disposition: His mother is advised to give him his asthma medication (albuterol) as instructed, give him acetaminophen for his fever, and have him checked today.

Most of the viruses that cause respiratory infections are more active during the autumn and spring (as well as winter), and they trigger asthma in asthmatic persons.

## CASE #15

EARLY SPRING                                                      TIME: 4:48AM

A three-month-old male infant

CC: Slight diarrhea

His mother states that the infant has had slight diarrhea, he has had three loose bowel movements but not a large amount. She denies any fever. He had been crying more, but he is asleep now. He has been feeding well and urinating a normal amount.

Disposition: His mother is advised to observe the infant. Three small loose bowel movements might be considered normal, especially in a breastfed infant.

## CASE #16

EARLY SPRING                                                      TIME: 7:30AM

A two-year-old male toddler

CC: Fever, ear-pulling, & a history of asthma

The child, a known asthmatic, has been sick for 5 days with fever and has been pulling on his ears.

Disposition: His mother is advised to give him his asthma medication (albuterol) as instructed, acetaminophen for fever, and to have him checked at the walk-in clinic today.

## CASE #17

A three-year-old female toddler

CC: Cough & wheezing
The child is an asthmatic and started to have a cough and wheezing today. Her asthma medication has just been started via the nebulizer today and she has a follow-up tomorrow.

Disposition: Her mother is advised to keep giving the asthma medications as instructed and to observe. If the child is getting better, then she may continue the medication (for cough, wheezing, shortness of breath or chest tightness) until she is better and keep giving the treatment around the clock every 4 hours. If she needs the treatment sooner than that, then she is to please call back. Once the child is getting better in a few days, then the albuterol can be given every 6 hours. She should continue to give the albuterol until the child's cough resolves completely. Also, the mother is to keep the appointment for asthma follow-up as previously scheduled for the morning. However, if any signs of respiratory distress are present or if the child is worsening or not responding to medication, she can be seen in the ED.

## CASE #18

A two-year-old male toddler

CC: Fever & diarrhea
The child received a Penicillin injection about two or three days ago, and now has a fever and diarrhea today.

Disposition: The mother is advised to give him acetaminophen for fever, and fluids. Dietary advice given regarding the diarrhea (avoid dairy, push starches, push fluid) and mother is asked to observe the child. The mother is advised to stop the milk and give him Pedialyte and other clear fluid, offer him foods like rice, applesauce, and plain yogurt, saltine crackers, graham crackers, and later chicken or turkey breast.

## CASE #19

TIME: 7:52PM

A 10-month-old female infant

CC: Burn
Her mother states that the infant just grabbed a bowl of the warm soup and she has a burn with redness on her left arm. There are no blisters. The burn is small and not circumferential (does not go around the arm in a circle).
Disposition: Her mother is advised to wash the area with cool water, put a cold compress on the red area, apply Bacitracin ointment (double antibiotic) twice a day, and observe. She may be checked in the clinic tomorrow if required.

## CASE #20

EARLY SPRING TIME: 5:00PM

A one-year-old male infant

CC: Diarrhea & cold symptoms
The infant has been having diarrhea and cold symptoms since yesterday. There has been no fever nor any difficulty breathing. The urine output has been normal.
Disposition: The mother is advised to give the infant Pedialyte and clear fluid, and then to keep him on a diet for diarrhea as instructed (soft, well-cooked rice, banana, applesauce and plain yogurt, and saltine and graham crackers). Also, use a humidifier, Normal Saline nose drops, and observe. The child is to be checked in the morning if required

## CASE #21

EARLY SPRING TIME: 8:16PM

An eight-month-old female infant

CC: Fever & whitish spots in the mouth
Her mother states that the infant had a fever a few days ago and that today she has developed some whitish spots in her mouth.
Disposition: Her mother is advised to give the infant enough fluid and have her checked tomorrow at the clinic.

The infant may have oral thrush or perhaps a viral infection. Given the history of fever, it is better to have the baby checked and receive a prescription for an appropriate medication at the clinic in the morning if need be.

## Case #22

A 19-day-old male neonate

CC: Cold symptoms
His mother states that the infant has a cold. He was seen by a physician yesterday and the use of Normal Saline nose drops were advised. His mother states the baby's temperature taken by an oral pacifier thermometer reveals 99.3ºF (37.3ºC) and that he is otherwise fine. I recommended that she take a rectal temperature and explained that we consider fever to be a temperature of 100.4ºF (38.0ºC) and higher.
Disposition: She is advised to please take a rectal temperature and if the child has a true fever then to call us back as the baby would require a septic work-up in the ED. A humidifier can also be used now.

## Case #23
Late autumn                                                     Time: 9:42PM

A five-month-old male infant

CC: Diarrhea
His mother states that the infant has had three watery stool today. He has been cranky and is rubbing his nose. He had a temperature of 101-102.0ºF (38.3-38.8ºC) for two days which has since subsided.
Disposition: His mother is advised to give the baby Pedialyte instead of formula for 12-24 hours (not for a longer period, as there are no nutrients in Pedialyte and too much Pedialyte can prolong diarrhea); she is then to offer him Lactose-free formula and to observe. The infant may be examined if he continues having diarrhea, if he is not urinating every 6-8 hours, if there is blood in the diarrhea, or if having severe abdominal pain (drawing legs up and continued crankiness).

# Case #24

A five-year-old female child

CC: Cough

Her mother states that the child has been coughing for two days; she has not had any fever and has no history of asthma. She was given some antihistamine cough syrup but she still coughs a great deal.

Disposition: Her mother is advised to give her warm steam exposure, or to use a humidifier in her room. She should offer her warm fluid to drink, and have the child checked tomorrow.

It is not advisable for children 6 years and under to be given over-the-counter cough and cold medication.

# Case #25

A five-week-old female neonate

CC: Fever

The infant started to have a fever since 3:00AM today. Her temperature is 102.9°F (39.3°C) and she has been constipated for one day.

Disposition: The mother is advised to take the infant to the ED to be checked as soon as possible.

A neonate (infant under 6-8 weeks of age) with any fever should be checked as soon as possible to rule out sepsis.

# Case #26

A three-year-old female toddler

CC: Swollen & itchy eyes

The child has been having swollen and itchy eyes for 2-3 days.

Her mother was giving her Dimetapp and Benadryl syrup but she is not getting better and she still has the problem.

Disposition: Her mother is advised to take the child to the walk-in clinic today to be checked. The daytime calls afford us more opportunities to go to the clinics versus ED and for the child to be checked and treated. There are eye drops containing antihistamine and mast cell stabilizers that help allergic conjunctivitis. However, an infection must also be ruled out.

## CASE #27

MID-SPRING                                                    TIME: 6:44PM

A five-year-old female child

CC: Congested eyes
The child has been having congested (red) eyes for one or two days. The mother denies any other problems.
Disposition: The mother is advised to wash the eyes with cool sterile water every 2-3 hours, and to take the child in to be checked tomorrow if she continues to have the problem.

## CASE #28

MID-SPRING                                                    TIME: 4:00AM

A seven-year-old female child

CC: Headache
The child has been having a headache since last night, she has no fever. She was not given any medication for her headache.
Disposition: Her father is advised to give her ibuprofen 200mg and to observe. She may be checked in the clinic today if her condition is not getting better.

## CASE #29

MID-SPRING                                                    TIME: 6:00PM

A 14-month-old female child

CC: Fever
The answering call service states that they have been told that the child had a fever, a temperature of 104.0°F (40.0°C). Her caregiver was called and a message was left to get back in-touch to receive the doctor's advice.
Disposition: It appears that the caregiver had left to take the child to the hospital and

so was not reached.

It is unclear without the history if the ED was advisable, as fever may be an indication that there is infection but not dangerous in and of itself. However, children 2 years and under with fevers ≥102.2-102.5ºF (39.0-39.1ºC) should be examined to make sure no serious bacterial infections are present and so visiting the ED may have ultimately been advised for this toddler.

## Case #30

Mid-spring                                                                Time: 6:00PM

A two-year-old male toddler

CC: Itchy eyes
His mother states that the child has been having itchy eyes. He had been seen at the clinic by the physician and received eye drops and he is getting better, but she has been using the eye drops less often.
Disposition: The mother is advised that it is acceptable to reduce the frequency of using the eye drops when the condition is improving, but that she should stay within the range which is instructed and complete the course of drops as directed.

## Case #31

Mid-winter                                                                Time: 9:15PM

A four-year-old female child

CC: Human bite, no broken skin
The child has been bitten by a three-year-old child at her grandmother's house. Her mother states there is some redness on the site of the bite (bite mark), the skin is not broken and is intact.
Disposition: Her mother is advised to use an ice pack on the affected area. Preventive measures are advised.
Given that there is no break in the skin, the child does not need to be seen, if no signs of infection (redness, worsening pain, swelling, etc.) ensue.

## Case #32

Mid-winter                                                                Time: 2:21AM

An eleven-year-old male child

CC: Pain in one thigh

The child complains of pain in his left thigh. His mother states that the child has a history of a head trauma when he was four years old and has had hemiparesis and some neurological problems secondary to his head injury. She states he develops pain sometimes. She also mentions that ibuprofen has been tried and it appears to be helping. The child is not in distress.

Disposition: His mother is advised regarding the use of ibuprofen every 6-8 hours for pain and to observe. If the condition persists, he may be examined at the walk-in clinic. The child might have paresthesia or neurologically-mediated pain but other problems such as joint, muscle, bone, and soft tissue pathological conditions should be considered and ruled out.

## Case #34

Mid-winter                                                          Time: 3:31AM

A two-year-old female toddler

CC: Diarrhea & vomiting

The child has diarrhea and vomiting which started about ten hours ago. There is no blood in either, and the vomit is not dark green colored (not bilious, that is).

Disposition: Her mother is advised to start oral electrolyte solution (Pedialyte) for her, which is to be given in small amounts, even by a syringe or spoon, and frequently. She may have 1 teaspoon (5mL) a minute for 12 consecutive minutes (2 oz.). Mother is to make sure she can retain it. In case she cannot retain the Pedialyte, she should be seen at the ED.

Otherwise, keep her on Pedialyte by giving sips as directed every 20 minutes until there has been no vomiting for 4 hours. At that point, solid foods can be reintroduced. She may have Pedialyte for twelve to twenty-four hours alone only, as there are no nutrients in the Pedialyte. Dietary advice regarding diarrhea (saltine crackers, graham crackers, soft rice, bread, non-buttered noodles, applesauce, banana, and plain yogurt) is given and the child is to be followed-up. If she is urinating every 6-8 hours, there is no blood in the stool, there are no severe pains, and there are improving symptoms (diarrhea <8-10 days), then it is okay to watch at home.

## Case #34

Mid-winter                                                          Time: 6:36AM

A five-year-old male preschool child

CC: Crankiness, possible earache
His mother states that the child has been cranky today. His brother has the same problem and he also has an earache.
Disposition: His mother is advised to give him acetaminophen and have him checked at the walk-in clinic today. When both children in one family have an earache, there is a strong possibility of an infection, either of viral or bacterial origin. Both children should be checked and receive appropriate treatments.

## Case #35
Mid-winter                                              Time: 6:46AM

A seven-year-old male child

CC: Earache
The child complains of ear pain.
Disposition: His mother is advised to give him acetaminophen (160mg/5mL) or ibuprofen (100mg/5mL), and to have him examined at the walk-in clinic today.

## Case #36
Mid-summer                                             Time: 12:59AM

A three-year-old female toddler

CC: Skin infection & fever
Her mother states that the child has a skin infection on her left arm. She has been having a fever since yesterday. The mother has been cleaning the area on her left arm and giving her Tylenol for the fever, but the child still has a high fever and a red, hot area on her left arm.
Disposition: The mother is advised to take the child in to be examined as soon as possible. The child should be examined and receive proper antibiotics. Cultures from blood and the skin lesion should be taken to determine the responsible organism, since some strains of bacteria such as MRSA (Methicillin-Resistant Staph-Aureus) are hard to treat and are multidrug resistant.

## Case #37
Mid-summer                                             Time: 9:37PM

A three-year-old female toddler

CC: Insect bite
Her mother states that the child appears to have an insect bite to the back of her leg. There is redness and swelling.
Disposition: The mother is advised to apply cold compresses on that area, use Calamine lotion and give her a dose of Benadryl and observe.
It is emphasized that mother should help the child to keep the skin clean and prevent infection. For pain, worsening redness, swelling, or new fever, the child should be checked.

## Case #38
Mid-summer                                                    Time: 10:20PM

A three-month-old male infant

CC: Nasal congestion
His mother states that the infant has had a cold for two days.
He has been having nasal congestion; there has been no fever.
Disposition: The mother is advised to use Normal Saline nose drops (1-2 drops into each nostril, 3-4 times per day for 3-5 days) and to observe. For fever, poor feeding or worsening symptoms, the infant should be checked.

## Case #39
Mid-summer                                                     Time: 7:26PM

A nine-year-old female child

CC: Earache
 Her mother states that the child has an earache. She has had no fevers. She was seen by a physician two days ago, and is taking Cephalexin every six hours, but she could not obtain the Pedi-otic ear drops from the Pharmacy as they did not have it in stock.
Disposition: The mother is advised to give her ibuprofen every six to eight hours, for the pain and to observe. Also, a call to the pharmacy will be made for a substitution. The child should be getting better in the next day or so, as antibiotics usually take 2-3 days to work. She should call again if she has any questions or if the child is not improving, and may be rechecked at that time if need be.

## Case #40

Mid-summer

Time: 8:32PM

This is regarding the previous case.
The pharmacist called and stated that they have Cortisporin ear drops in-stock that maybe substituted for the Pedi-otic ear drops.

## Case #41

Mid-summer

Time: 4:35PM

A two-year-old female toddler

CC: Nasal congestion & nosebleed
The child has had nasal congestion and nose bleeding once yesterday and once today.
Disposition: The mother is advised to use Neosynephrine nose drops, one drop into each of her nostrils, and Bacitracin ointment is to be applied with Q-tips in her nose, and to have the child examined tomorrow in the clinic. Alternatively, she may use Nasal Saline spray and Vaseline at the nares to add moisture to the area so that dry mucus does not occur, leading to bleeding.

## Case #42

Mid-summer

Time: 5:15PM

An 18-month-old female toddler

CC: High fever
 The answering service relayed that the mother called and states that the child has been having a high fever for two days. I tried to get in touch with them and the answering service also tried calling them, but there was no response.
Disposition: It appears they left to take the child to the ED.
Again, while a fever in and of itself is not dangerous, a high fever (>102.2-102.5°F [39.0-39.1°C]) must be taken seriously in a child less than 3 year of age, as they are at risk for serious bacterial infections like urinary tract infections and blood infections.

## Case #43

Mid-summer

Time: 6:50PM

A 17-year-old adolescent female

CC: Abdominal pain

The adolescent has been having abdominal pain and had been seen at the ED twice within the past few days. She states she has a pain in the right lower part of her abdomen that has been progressive and that it now hurts when she moves or jumps up and down.

Disposition: Given the severity, location and progression of the pain, she is advised to be reevaluated at ED.

Abdominal pain which gets worse with movement is suggestive of an organic condition and should be checked in a timely manner.

## CASE #44

MID-SUMMER                                              TIME: 5:27PM

A one-month-old male neonate

CC: Foaming at the mouth

His father states that the infant has had some foam in his mouth, it just happened after feeding and he has since coughed.

Disposition: The father is advised regarding the baby's color and breathing. He should make sure the infant is generally  well and that is he is breathing well with clearly patent (open) airways. Gastroesophageal (GE) reflux precautions are given (hold baby upright for 20 minutes after each feeding, burp more frequently after each one oz., create an incline by placing a towel or sheet under the crib mattress so that the baby's head is always higher than his bottom and likewise give him smaller more frequent feedings). Nasal Saline drops may be used to make sure the nasal passages are open. The neonate should be evaluated at the ED if the baby is in any distress or if he were to develop a cough, or if it happens again.

## CASE #45

EARLY SUMMER                                            TIME: 8:21PM

A nine-month-old male infant

CC: Ear infection

The infant has an ear infection now and is on an antibiotic. His mother states that the infant coughs and vomits after coughing. She is requesting cough syrup. The infant has no history of asthma.

Disposition: The mother is advised to offer the infant clear fluid and, when she feeds him, to give him a smaller amount in shorter intervals so he can retain the fluid better.

She is advised that over-the-counter cough syrup is not recommended for infants. She should observe and take the infant for follow- up if he is not improving after more than 2- 3 days on the antibiotics. If he is not improving, then the ears should be rechecked as the ear infection might not be responding to the antibiotic (the antibiotic might not have been strong enough).

## CASE #46

EARLY SUMMER                                           TIME: 2:07PM

A nine-month-old male infant
CC: Ear infection
The mother states that the infant has an ear infection and has been on antibiotic (Amoxicillin). He vomited the medicine today.
Disposition: The mother is advised regarding giving him clear fluid and to later retry giving the medicine, little by little, by aiming for the pocket between his cheek and gums. She is to offer him water after giving the medicine. She should observe the infant and call us back if needed.

## CASE #47

EARLY SUMMER                                           TIME: 5:00PM

A three-year-old male child
CC: Fever
The answering service states that the child had a fever today. He had a temperature 102.0°F (38.8°C). The telephone number that was given was tried and it was a wrong number.
Unfortunately, there are calls where the physician cannot reach the caregiver. This is also, is a part of the off-hours experience and the on-call physician should be familiar with this issue, and take notes documenting the attempts to contact the family.

## CASE #48

EARLY SUMMER                                           TIME: 6:19AM

A six-month-old male infant

CC: Fever, cold for more than one week
The infant has a fever. His temperature is 102.9°F (39.3°C) today. He has been having a cold for more than one week.

Disposition: His mother is advised to give him acetaminophen and to observe. If he continues to have a fever despite antipyretic, then he is to be examined at the ED today, as it is the weekend and so the clinic is closed. The infant that has a cold that is lasting more than one week and now is associated with a new, high fever, should be checked as there may be a secondary bacterial infection like pneumonia (lung infection), otitis media (ear infection), or a sinus infection present.

## CASE #49

EARLY SUMMER                                                          TIME: 11:40PM

An 18-month-old female toddler

CC: Ingestion, one sunflower seed
The mother states that the child swallowed one sunflower seed, and vomited after that. There appears to be a streak of blood in the vomitus along with the seed.
Disposition: The mother is advised to make sure the child is breathing well, to give her some water to drink, and to observe. The mother may get back in-touch in case any further problems should arise.

## CASE #50

EARLY SUMMER                                                          TIME: 7:12PM

A four-week-old male neonate

CC: Constipation, crankiness, & one episode of vomiting
The infant has had no bowel movements today. He has been cranky and vomited once. There was no blood nor dark green material (bile) in the vomit. He is asleep now.
Disposition: The mother is advised to observe the neonate. In case of continued crankiness and vomiting, or if not urinating at least once every 6 hours, then the neonate is to be examined at a hospital ED.

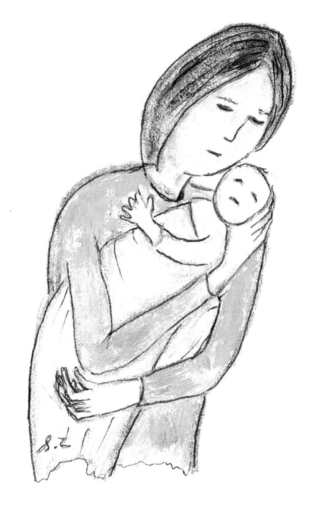

Case #25

A Neonate with fever

# Chapter Two

Case #51

Early summer                                                    Time: 6:00PM

A seven-month-old female infant

CC: Ear discharge, fever & vomiting
The infant has been having secretions from her right ear for about four days. She has not been seen by a physician. She now has a fever and vomiting today.
Disposition: The mother is advised to take the infant to be checked tonight as the infant has signs of otitis media with perforation of the eardrum and should be checked and receive proper antibiotics sooner rather than later, given the young age and the duration of ongoing symptoms without treatment.

Case #52

Early summer                                                    Time: 9:58PM

A six-year-old female child

CC: Hives
The child has developed hives since yesterday. Her mother does not know if she was exposed to anything specific. There are no new exposures to foods and the child is otherwise well, without any respiratory symptoms. She takes no medications.
Disposition: The mother is advised to give her Benadryl and observe. She is to avoid giving her hyper-allergenic foods like eggs, chocolate, seafood, peanuts, strawberry, tomato sauce, and whatever she suspects the child may have been allergic to. Very often

urticaria may be nonspecific and the cause might not be elucidated. She may get back in touch if she has any further questions.

## CASE #53

EARLY SUMMER                                                            TIME: 8:36PM

A two-month-old male infant

CC: Slight cough

The infant has been having a slight cough for two days, he has no fever and has been feeding well.

Disposition: His mother is advised to use Normal Saline nose drops (1-2 drops into his nostrils 3-4 times per day for 3-5 days) to wash out the mucus. She is to make sure the infant is taking the formula and may give him smaller amounts of formula, and feed him in shorter intervals, to prevent vomiting. A humidifier can also be used. If his cough persists, he may be examined tomorrow, given his young age.

## CASE #54

EARLY SUMMER                                                            TIME: 12:04AM

A three-year-old male toddler

CC: Diarrhea

The child has been having watery stool for two days. He had been vomiting yesterday. The vomit had no blood and was not bilious (not dark green). He has not had any vomiting today, but he still has watery stool.

Disposition: The mother is advised to give him Pedialyte and make sure he can retain the Pedialyte. A bland diet consisting of saltine crackers, graham crackers, rice, bread, and banana may also be given. Avoid dairy except for plain yogurt for a couple days. If he looks weak, or the condition persists and he is unable to tolerate fluids, or if he is not voiding, then he may be seen at the ED.

## CASE #55

EARLY SUMMER                                                            TIME: 5:50PM

A two-year-old male toddler

CC: Fever & exposure to a cousin with bacteremia

His mother states that the child had an ear infection a few days ago; he was seen by the physician and has been on Amoxicillin. He currently has a fever with a temperature 103.0°F (39.4°C). According to his mother, the child was exposed to his cousin who was hospitalized and was found out to have Strep pneumonia bacteremia.

Disposition: His mother is advised to give the child Tylenol (160mg/5mL) and have him evaluated at the hospital, given a failure to respond to oral medication and the exposure to a cousin with bacteremia.

## CASE #56

EARLY SUMMER                                                    TIME: 5:50AM

A two-year-old male toddler

CC: Fever & greenish nasal discharge

The child has been having a fever for about four days. He has been coughing and having yellowish-greenish discharge from his nose. He was seen by a physician before, and no antibiotic was given. His temperature is 101.8°F (38.7°C) this morning.

Disposition: His mother prefers that he be reexamined today. The mother is advised to take him to be reexamined later today at clinic, as per her preference.

## CASE #57

EARLY SUMMER                                                    TIME: 9:50AM

A seven-year-old female child

CC: Hyperactivity

The mother complains that the child is hyperactive and acting out today. Also, the mother needs a prescription for Propranolol tablets for herself.

Disposition: The mother is advised that as a pediatrician I cannot refill her medication and that she should please contact her own physician regarding the medicine. As far as the child's behavioral concerns, as it is not an urgent matter, she can make an appointment on a weekday to discuss these issues with her child's pediatrician.

## CASE #58

EARLY SUMMER                                                    TIME: 10:21AM

A 22-day-old female neonate

CC: Crying at night & possible noisy breathing

Her mother states the infant has been crying at night for the last two nights, and is possibly having noisy breathing. The infant had been examined a few days ago, and was fine.

Disposition: The mother is advised regarding crying and to observe the baby for any breathing problem or feeding problem and to have her reexamined if needed. Nasal Saline can be tried to see if the noise dissipates with that intervention. If there is difficulty with breathing or feeding, the baby can be reexamined.

## CASE #59

EARLY SUMMER                                          TIME: 4: 37PM

A two-year-old male toddler

CC: Hemoglobinopathy & fever
The child has a hemoglobinopathy (β-thalassemia-sickle cell disease). He has been having a fever today, and his temperature is not coming down with Tylenol. He has been hospitalized several times.

Disposition: His mother is advised to give him more fluid and hydrate him well and to take him to the hospital. The above child with compound hemoglobinopathy (β-thalassemia-sickle cell disease) must be treated like those with sickle cell disease who, when developing fever should be seen promptly to receive IV fluids for pain crises and antibiotics for occult bacteremia, as they are at increased risk for bacterial infection. A blood culture should be done prior to the initiation of treatment to determine the offending bacteria.

## CASE #60

EARLY SUMMER                                          TIME: 10:55PM

A two-year-old female toddler

CC: Cardiac problem & low oxygen saturation
The child is connected to a ventilator at a facility. She has an underlying cardiac problem. She is on potassium, Lasix, Flovent, and albuterol. The nurse states that the child has a rapid pulse with low oxygen saturation (SpO2). The nurse does not know any details about the cardiac condition of the child.

Disposition: She is advised to consult the physician on site at the facility and that the child should receive oxygen if the oxygen saturation is less than 90-92%, if the low SpO2 is a new finding. If there is no on-site physician, then 911 can be called to evaluate the child in-person.

## Case #61

A four-year-old male child

CC: Bumps to the back of the throat & a chronic hoarse voice
The mother states the child has some bumps to the back of his throat. He has been having a hoarse voice for a long time. She denies his having any fever, vomiting or any other problem.
Disposition: The mother is advised to make an appointment for the child to be examined later, in the day ahead. Since the condition has been ongoing and the child is not in any distress, it is not necessary that the child be seen at the ED now. The child may be examined at the clinic when it opens later today.

## Case #62

A six-month-old female infant

CC: Cough
Her mother states the infant has been having a cough for two days. She denies having any fever and vomiting. She has no history of asthma/wheezing. Her mother has been giving her an OTC medicine, Pediacare.
Disposition: The mother is advised to use Normal Saline nose drops (1-2 drops into the nostrils, 3-4 times per day for 3-5 days), give her more fluid and observe. She may be checked tomorrow. Over-the-counter cold and cough syrup is not recommended at this age, so she should stop giving the Pediacare.

## Case #63

A one-year-old male infant

CC: Possible "dislocation of the shoulder"
The mother states the child was with his eleven-year-old brother and was pulled up by his arm, he started to cry and he appears to have a dislocation of his shoulder. He is asleep now.

Disposition: The mother is advised that if the child is not moving his arm/not using his arm, then he is to be examined.

There could be a possible dislocation at the elbow, commonly referred to as a Nursemaid's elbow, which can easily be reduced by a physician.

## CASE #64

A 13-year-old male adolescent

CC: Puncture wound, with the tip of a pencil
The teen's grandmother states that he accidentally punctured the sole of his foot with the tip of a pencil.
Disposition: The grandmother and the adolescent boy were advised to clean the area with the soap and water, apply a warm compress and double antibiotic ointment and observe.
He may be seen tomorrow if required (pain, worry for foreign body retention).

## CASE #65

A two-month-old male infant

CC: Tiny bloody mucus on diaper
His mother states that a tiny bloody mucus was seen in his diaper. He has normal bowel movement with no diarrhea. He does not have any sign of bleeding and he is otherwise healthy.
Disposition: His mother is advised to observe and have the baby examined tomorrow in clinic. The mother should save the diaper with the bloody mucus, to show the healthcare provider.

## CASE #66

A three-year-old female toddler

CC: Diarrhea
The child has developed diarrhea today. She has been having watery stools. There have

been four such episodes. She has not had any vomiting. She is drinking Pedialyte well, urinating normally and has a normal activity level.

Disposition: The mother is advised to keep her on Pedialyte and clear fluid as long as she is without vomiting and to introduce solids soon. Dietary advice regarding diarrhea (white rice, applesauce, banana, plain yogurt, saltine and graham crackers) is given. She already has an appointment scheduled, and is to be checked tomorrow.

## CASE #67

EARLY WINTER                                                        TIME: 10:11PM

A two-week-old male neonate

CC: Constipation
The answering service reveals that the infant has constipation.
There was no response when the mother was called. Perhaps there had been infrequent stools and then the neonate probably had a bowel movement. At this age, the consistency of the stool is more important than the stool frequency. If the stools are soft and semisolid, and not hard little balls/ hard pellet-like stools, then going a couple days without a bowel movement is not considered constipation.

## CASE #68

EARLY WINTER                                                        TIME: 12: 35AM

A two-year-old female toddler

CC: Fever
The child has a fever; her temperature is 101.8°F (38.7°C). She was seen by a physician today, and the mother has been told she has a viral infection. Her mother is concerned because despite giving her ibuprofen about an hour ago, her temperature is not coming down.
Disposition: Her mother is advised to give her more fluid and to observe. She can also try Tylenol. If she continues to be febrile despite these measures and she looks sicker, then she can be reexamined at the ED.

## CASE #69

EARLY WINTER                                                        TIME: 3:50AM

A six-month-old female infant

CC: Cough & slight fever

The infant has been coughing for two days and has been having a slight fever. The mother had called last night and was given advice. One dose of Tylenol was given about six hours ago.

Disposition: Her mother is advised to give her another dose of Tylenol (may be given every 4-6 hours for fever, temperature ≥ 100.4°F [38.0°C]) and offer her more fluid (water, juice) and to have her checked at the clinic this morning, given the child's young age.

## CASE #70

EARLY WINTER                                            TIME: 4:30AM

A two-year-old male toddler

CC: High fever

The child currently has a temperature of 104.0°F (40.0°C). He was seen at the ED two days ago. The mother was told that he has a viral infection. His mother is giving him Motrin and Tylenol as instructed, but the toddler continues to have high fevers.

Disposition: His mother is advised to give him Motrin (100 mg/5mL), for a temperature ≥100.4°F (38.0°C) and to offer him more fluid (juice, soup, ginger ale). She is to have him reexamined at the pediatric clinic today, given the height and duration of the fever.

## CASE #71

Late winter                                             Time: 7:28PM

A three-month-old male infant

CC: Excessive crying & vomiting

The infant has been crying excessively for the last two or three hours and he has been vomiting. These symptoms are new. He has had no recent bowel movements.

Disposition: The mother is advised to take the infant to the ED so that he may be examined.

An infant with excessive crying should be examined urgently.

## CASE #72

Late winter                                             Time: 1:25AM

A three-year-old male toddler

CC: Abdominal pain

The child has been having abdominal pain around the umbilical area off and on for two days. There is no right lower quadrant pain. He has no vomiting. He did have a fever at the onset of his symptoms, which has since subsided.

Disposition: The mother is advised to have the child examined tomorrow. Periumbilical pain that is not consistent is usually a sign of functional rather than organic origin, unless it travels to the right lower quadrant, in that case the mother is advised to seek care sooner.


## CASE #73

Late winter                                                    Time: 5:35PM

A two-year-old male toddler

CC: Fever & cold/cough in a patient with a history of asthma

The child has been having a fever for two days. His temperature is around 101.0°F (38.3°C). He has a runny nose and a cough. He has a history of bronchial asthma. Tylenol was given for his fever.

Disposition: His father is advised to give him more fluid (juice, soup, ginger ale) to drink and to start his asthma medication (albuterol) as instructed and observe. He may be checked tomorrow if there is no respiratory distress overnight.


## CASE #74

Late winter                                                    Time: 4:18PM

An eight-year-old female child

CC: Fever

The child has been having a fever for three days. She was seen at the ED last night and a throat culture was taken. Her temperature is 100.0°F (37.7°C) today.

Disposition: The mother is advised to give her Tylenol (160 mg/5mL) for her fever/sore throat and to observe the child and follow-up on the report of the throat culture.


## CASE #75

LATE WINTER                                                    TIME: 1:59PM

A three-year-old male toddler

CC: Cold & asthma, needs medication (refill request)

The child has a cold and started to have wheezing.

The mother states the child needs albuterol inhalation solution and Normal Saline inhalation solution for the nebulizer.

Disposition: His medications were ordered directly to the pharmacy of choice by telephone, and his mother was advised regarding their use (the albuterol to be used every four hours in the beginning until his cough is much better, for about 5 days and then every six hours and continue until he has no cough at all, not even when he runs). She is to have him use the medicine as instructed and observe. Please keep his asthma follow-up appointment.

## CASE #76

LATE WINTER                                                        TIME: 7:47AM

A 15-month-old male toddler

CC: Vomiting & possible fever

The child has vomited twice today and has a subjective fever.

His temperature has not been taken.

Disposition: His mother is advised to take his temperature and give him clear fluid and Pedialyte and observe, she is to get back in touch if required.

## CASE #77

LATE WINTER                                                        TIME: 9:59AM

A five-month-old male infant

CC: Diarrhea

The infant has been having diarrhea twice since last night. He has had no vomiting and his temperature was taken in his axilla and is 99.7°F (37.6°C).

Disposition: His mother is advised that the infant is to be observed. In case of frequent loose bowel movements, the mother should stop the formula and offer him Pedialyte for about twelve hours. Thereafter, she can also give a Lactose-free (Lactofree formula) if the Pedialyte is well tolerated.

## CASE #78

LATE WINTER                                                        TIME: 10:42AM

A two-week-old female infant

CC: Question regarding medication
The neonate is on Phenobarbital. Her mother had a question regarding how to give the medicine to the baby.
Disposition: The mother was instructed on how to measure the medication accurately by using a small syringe. She may then give it to the infant from one side of her mouth, between her cheek and gums and offer a small amount of water (either boiled cool water, filtered, or bottled water for infants) right after the medicine is given. She is to keep her appointment for follow-up.

## CASE #79

A five-month-old male

CC: Diarrhea & possible fever
The mother had called previously regarding the infant who had diarrhea and a probable fever. She had a question about how to take the temperature.
Disposition: The mother is advised to get an axillary thermometer and use it at the armpit and to give him Infants' Tylenol every 4-6 hours for a temperature ≥100.4°F (38.0°C).
Taking the rectal temperature is indeed more accurate, but in this case of diarrhea and with the possibility of rectal irritation in infants, an axillary temperature may be preferable. If the temperature is ≥102.2-102.5°F (39.0C-39.1°C), then it is best that the child be checked.

## CASE #80

A five-month-old male infant

CC: How to take the infant's temperature with diarrhea?
The mother had called shortly before and needed clarificationas she had been advised that a rectal temperature is the most accurate method in a baby under 6 months. She is indeed correct; however, an exception can be made in the face of diarrhea, given the presence of rectal irritation.
Mom called again regarding the temperature and needed more instruction. The mother was told that because of the diarrhea, taking rectal temperature was not advised

to prevent further irritation. She also needed to know what constitutes a temperature and so was told that temperature up to 100.4°F is normal. Again, if there is a fever ≥102.2-102.5°F (39.0-39.1°C) then the baby can be seen at the clinic.

## CASE #81

LATE WINTER                                                    TIME: 1:00AM

A ten-year-old male child

CC: Sore throat, cough, a lump on the neck & a history of asthma
The mother states that the child is complaining of a sore throat. He has been coughing today, and he feels a lump on his neck. He has history of asthma.
Disposition: His mother is advised to give him Children's Tylenol (160mg/5mL) every 4-6 hours or Children's Motrin (100mg/5mL) every 6-8 hours for his fever, and to start to use his asthma medication (albuterol) for his cough. Also, she is to have him gargle with warm salty water. She is to take him to the clinic to have a throat culture later today.

## CASE #82

LATE WINTER                                                    TIME: 4:30AM

A 21-month-old female toddler

CC: Vomiting
The toddler has vomited today twice after taking orange juice. She has neither fever nor any other problem.
Disposition: Her mother is advised to give her Pedialyte in small amounts (sips) and to observe. If she cannot retain the Pedialyte at all, then she may be seen at the Emergency Department.

## CASE #83

LATE WINTER                                                    TIME: 7:57AM

A two-year-old male toddler

CC: Ear infection
His mother states that the child has been having an ear infection, and he is on Amoxicillin 250mg per teaspoon, and taking half a teaspoon (125mg) three times per day. However, it appears he still has a problem.

Disposition: The mother is advised to increase the dose of medication (to one teaspoon three times per day) and to observe, if he keeps having a problem and fever, then the medication is to be changed.

The recommended dose of Amoxicillin for the treatment of acute otitis media is 80-90mg/kg per day divided in two or three doses. If a child does not respond when on a good dose of a proper antibiotic after 2-3 days, then the ear should be rechecked as a stronger antibiotic may be needed.

## Case #84

Late winter                                                                 Time: 8:25AM

A six-week-old female neonate

CC: Cold symptoms, no fever
The infant has cold symptoms with no fever.
Disposition: The mother is advised to use Normal Saline nose drops (one or two drops in the nostrils, three or four times per day for 3-5 days), to use a humidifier in the room, and to observe. The infant may be examined if she has any fever (rectal temperature of ≥100.4ºF [38.0ºC]).

## Case #85

Late winter                                                                 Time: 9:16AM

A nine-month-old male infant

CC: Crankiness while being treated for an ear infection
His mother states that the infant has been on Amoxicillin for an ear infection and it appears that he is getting better and has no fever, but that he has been gagging on the formula and has been cranky.
Disposition: The mother is advised to observe the infant. If the infant is vomiting or continues to be fussy, then she is to have him rechecked.

## Case #86

Late winter                                                                 Time: 9:16AM

A six-month-old female infant

CC: Fever & cough, vomited phlegm

The infant has a temperature of 101.0ºF (38.3ºC) with cough. She vomited phlegm twice today.

Disposition: The mother is advised to give her Infants' Tylenol every 4-6 hours for fever, (temperature ≥ 100.4ºF [38.0ºC]), to use Normal Saline nose drops (1-2 drops into the nostrils, 3-4 times per day for 3-5 days) to offer the baby more fluid (water, apple juice or white grape juice, and breastmilk or formula) and to observe. If the temperature is <102.2ºF (39.0ºC), then it is likely due to a viral infection. However, the infant may be examined if the condition persists.

## CASE #87
LATE WINTER                                                    TIME: 10:12AM

An eleven-year-old male child

CC: Fever & vomiting

The child has a fever and has been vomiting today. He received his immunization against Hepatitis B and Varicella yesterday.

Disposition: The mother is advised to give him Children's Tylenol (160 mg/5mL), every 4-6 hours or Children's Motrin (100mg/5mL), every 6-8 hours for his fever. She is to offer him Pedialyte and clear fluid (Gatorade, clear juice, ginger ale) and to observe. If the condition persists, then she is to take him to be checked. The fever and vomiting are not likely to be related to the immunizations, as vomiting is not a common side effect of vaccination. He has probably contracted a viral infection.

## CASE #88
LATE WINTER                                                    TIME: 10:52AM

A two-month-old male infant

CC: Concentrated formula given

The mother states that she gave the infant concentrated formula for two feedings by mistake. The baby appears to be fine now.

Disposition: The mother is advised to give him 4oz. of water to drink and to be careful in preparing the formula, giving him the regular strength of formula.

## CASE #89
LATE WINTER                                                    TIME: 11:09AM

A three-year-old female toddler

CC: Eye discharge, fever & swollen eyelids
The mother states that the child has been having eye discharge for three days. She had a fever last night. Her eyelids are swollen today.
Disposition: The mother is advised to have the child examined today. Also, she is advised to clean the eyes with sterile water, using cotton balls to carefully wipe the discharge from the eyelids.

## Case #90

Late winter                                                    Time: 12:08PM

A four-year-old female child

CC: Asthmatic & rapid heartbeat after using albuterol
Her mother states that the child is an asthmatic and that she is on prednisone and albuterol solution for inhalation 0.5mL via nebulizer. The medication is being used and the child appears to have a rapid heartbeat as a result.
Disposition: The mother is advised to decrease the dose of albuterol to 0.25mL and to skip a dose if the heartbeat is fast and observe.
A fast heart beat is a known side effect of albuterol. If the heartbeat normalizes, she can then go back to the regular dose thereafter.

## Case #91
Late winter                                                    Time: 12:30PM

A four-month-old male infant

CC: Hair loss
His mother is concerned regarding the hair loss.
Disposition: The mother is advised that hair loss, especially to the back of the scalp of an infant, is normal and that the hair will grow back. She is reassured. She should keep his appointment for his regular four-month-old check-up.

## Case #92
Late winter                                                    Time: 1:26PM

A five-year-old female child

CC: Flatulence (passes a great deal of gas)

The child had a stomach virus, and she was seen by a physician yesterday and the mother has been advised. Today, the child has a great deal of gas.

Disposition: The mother is advised to avoid offering the child cow's milk and dairy products for a few days, and to also avoid raw fruits and vegetables and beans for a few days after having diarrhea. Lactaid milk can be given for a week or so thereafter.

## CASE #93

LATE WINTER                                                    TIME: 4:24PM

A five-month-old female infant

CC: Mouth lesion

The infant has one mouth lesion and no fever.

Disposition: The mother is advised to offer the infant enough fluid (water, apple juice or white grape juice, formula or breast milk) and to keep her mouth clean and observe. The infant can be examined on Monday if required (weekend call).

## CASE #94

LATE WINTER                                                    TIME: 5:42PM

A 16-month-old female toddler

CC: Diarrhea & vomiting

The child has been having diarrhea for three days. She also vomited two days ago. She has loose stools three or four times per day. Her mother denies any blood or mucus in stool. There is no bile nor blood in the vomit. There has been no fever.

Disposition: The mother is advised to offer her Pedialyte and clear fluid (ginger ale, white grape juice, Jell-O) and then foods like rice, saltine crackers, applesauce, banana, and plain yogurt, and to observe.

## CASE #95

LATE WINTER                                                    TIME: 10:04PM

A five-month-old male infant

CC: Diarrhea & vomiting

The infant has diarrhea and vomiting that started today.

He has vomited twice today and has been having two or three very loose and watery stools today. There is neither blood nor mucus in stool, nor is there any blood nor bile in the vomit.

Disposition: The mother is advised to stop the formula and to offer the infant Pedialyte in small amounts frequently for about twelve to twenty-four hours and to then start lactose-free formula (Lactofree formula). The mother should have him examined if the infant cannot retain the Pedialyte or if the condition persists. Rotavirus infections are mostly active during the cooler seasons.

## Case #96

Late winter                                                                    Time: 5:35PM

An eight-month-old male infant

CC: Cold & fever

His mother states that the infant has been having a cold and fever for two to three days. He was seen by a physician and is on Dimetapp, but the infant has now developed ear discharge.

Disposition: The mother is advised to go to pharmacy and that I will start the child on Amoxicillin. He is to follow-up at the clinic tomorrow. Also, she is advised to clean the ear discharge with Hydrogen Peroxide (just the outer part) until the child's ear is checked the next day.

## Case #97

Late winter                                                                    Time: 6:08PM

A four-month-old male infant

CC: Diarrhea & vomiting

His mother states that the infant has been having diarrhea for three days. He vomited today and he has no fever. He was seen by a physician two days ago. The mother was advised to use Pedialyte and other dietary advice was given.

Disposition: The mother is advised to offer the Pedialyte in small amounts and to make sure that the infant can retain it. In case he cannot retain the Pedialyte, then he is to be seen at the ED. Breastmilk or Lactose-free formula can then be offered if the Pedialyte was well tolerated.

## Case #98

A six-week-old female neonate

CC: Rash

Her mother states that the baby has a minute pinkish rash on his forehead, face and neck. The mother denies any other problem. There is no fever, no change in feeding pattern, no change in voiding pattern, and there are no pustules nor dark redness to the rash.

Disposition: The mother is advised to bathe the baby more often and to pat her dry, and then use corn starch powder (not talc) with her hand (to avoid the baby inhaling the powder) at the neck area only. She also is advised to make sure the room temperature is appropriate for the baby and not to keep her too warm. She is to avoid overdressing the baby to prevent heat rash, and to observe. If there are no other symptoms, the baby can be checked in the clinic if there is no improvement. The mother is to call us if other symptoms were to develop.

## Case #99

A nine-year-old male child

CC: Chronic asthma & has run out of Singulair

The child has chronic asthma. He is on Singulair 5 mg tablet daily. He has run out the medication.

Disposition: His mother is advised to go to the pharmacy and the prescription will be given by phone.

Singulair (Leukotriene receptor antagonist; Montelukast) is to be continued for the prevention of chronic asthma and exercise induced bronchoconstriction. If no acute exacerbation, asthma and allergy medications can be refilled over the phone.

## Case #100

A 23-month-old female toddler

CC: Diarrhea & vomiting

The toddler has been having diarrhea and vomiting for two days. Pedialyte has been given.

Disposition: The caregiver is advised that in case the toddler cannot retain the Pedialyte, she is to be seen at the ED. Pedialyte should be given in small amounts frequently and when she can retain the Pedialyte, then one may offer her other clear fluid like ginger ale and white grape juice, and to also continue the Pedialyte. The caregiver is to avoid giving the toddler milk for a few days. When she has no vomiting, and is feeling better, then she may have white rice, applesauce, saltine crackers, banana, rice cereal and plain yogurt. In a few days, she may have a hard-boiled egg and well-cooked chicken or turkey breast. Rotavirus infections are more prevalent in daycare attendees. The caregiver should wash his or her hands after changing the diaper to prevent further spreading the virus.

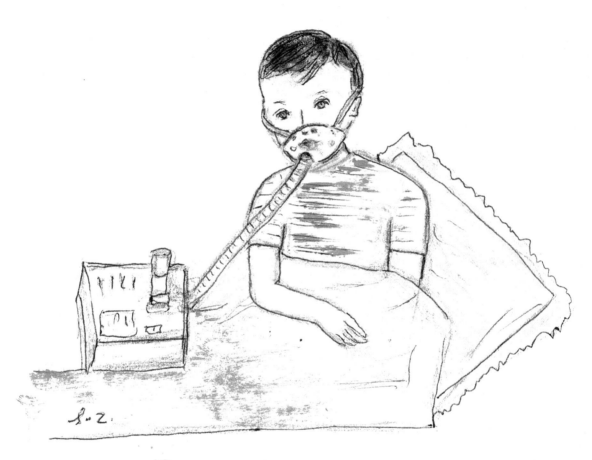

A Case of asthma

# CHAPTER THREE

## CASE #101

LATE WINTER                                      TIME: 6:58PM

A three-year-old male toddler

CC: Diarrhea & vomiting
The child has had non-bloody, non-mucoid diarrhea and non-bloody, non-bilious vomiting today.
Disposition: The caregiver is advised to start Pedialyte and clear fluid like ginger ale and white grape juice. When he has no more vomiting, he can then have white rice, applesauce, saltine crackers or graham crackers, banana, plain yogurt and more clear fluid. The caregiver is to avoid giving the toddler cow's milk and raw vegetables and fruits for a few days. If he cannot retain the Pedialyte, then he may be seen at the ED.

## CASE #102

LATE WINTER                                      TIME: 7:12PM

An eight-month-old female infant

CC: Ear infection
Her mother states that the infant has a history of having had a right ear infection one week ago. She was seen by a physician and she has been on Amoxicillin for one week. She is doing well, and she has neither fever nor other problem, but she is still touching her left ear.
Disposition: The mother is advised to finish the course of the antibiotic and observe

41

and keep the appointment for follow up in 1-3 weeks (2-4 weeks after the initiation of antibiotics).

There may be lingering serous fluid at this point causing the pain, but if the child is without fever and improved overall, then likely the infection is responding to the Amoxicillin. If the child were to have a fever or worsening symptoms, then she could be seen sooner than the scheduled follow-up.

## CASE #103
LATE WINTER                                              TIME: 10:19PM

An eleven-month-old male infant

CC: Vomiting
The mother states that the infant has vomited two or three times today. He has neither fever nor diarrhea. His vomitus is non- bilious (not green color).
Disposition: His mother is advised to give him Pedialyte in small amounts frequently and to observe the infant. Also, the mother is advised to make sure he can retain the Pedialyte. In case the infant keeps vomiting and cannot retain the Pedialyte, he may be seen at the ED.

## CASE #104
LATE WINTER                                              TIME: 10:55PM

A one-year-old female infant

CC: Vomiting
The mother states that the infant vomited twice today. There was no blood nor bile in the vomit. She has had no fever. Her bowel movements are normal.
Disposition: The mother is advised to start Pedialyte in small amounts and to observe. If the infant keeps vomiting and cannot retain the Pedialyte, then she may be seen at the ED.
Vomiting, if not related to a feeding problem, might have a viral origin and, during the wintertime, influenza and other respiratory viruses are among the responsible viruses.

## CASE #105
MID-SPRING                                               TIME: 5:00PM

A six-year-old male child

CC: Pink eyes

The child appears to have pinkish eyes, no discharge.

Disposition: His mother is advised to wash the eyes with cool water and to observe. At mid-spring time, pink eyes may usually be attributed to allergic conjunctivitis. Without discharge nor lash mattering, it can be observed, but should these occur, the mother should call again.

## CASE #106

MID-SPRING                                                                    TIME: 5:30PM

A four-month-old male infant

CC: Cough

The infant has been coughing for five days. He has no fever. He throws up after the cough sometimes. He has no history of asthma/wheezing.

Disposition: His mother is advised to use Normal Saline nose drops (1-2 drops into the nostrils, 3-4 times per day for 3-5 days) to wash out the mucus. She is to offer him fluid in small amounts and shorter intervals so he can retain the fluid and formula. She is to use a humidifier around the baby and to observe. If he were to develop a fever, or if the cold lasts more than one week and he is not improving by then, then she is to have the infant checked.

## CASE #107

MID-SPRING                                                                    TIME: 5:45PM

A three-year-old female toddler

CC: Fever, skin lesions & an exposure to chickenpox

The child has a fever and itchy skin lesions. She was exposed to chickenpox about one or two weeks ago.

Disposition: Her mother is advised to give her Children's Tylenol (160mg/5mL, 6mL every 4-6 hours) for fever and use Calamine lotion on the skin lesions and to keep the child at home and observe.

The incubation period of varicella infection (chickenpox) is about 10 days to 21 days after the exposure to the rash.

At the time of this call, the varicella immunization (chickenpox) was not yet available and so it was indeed a common virus among toddlers.

## CASE #108

MID-SPRING

A seven-year-old male child

CC: Medication refill request

The child has a history of Epilepsy and is on Tegretol tablets and he has run out of the medication. His mother states she was advised to get the brand name and not the generic and wants it to be ordered to the pharmacy.

Disposition: The medication is ordered. The mother is advised to please keep his follow-up appointment.

## CASE #109

MID-SPRING

A two-year-old female toddler

CC: Blisters in the mouth

The child appears to have some blisters in her mouth, mostly to the back of the throat.

Disposition: The mother is advised to keep the child's mouth clean and let her drink some water each time after she eats, and make sure she takes adequate fluid (juice, soup, ginger ale) and offer her soft and mild food. In case of fever, mother may give her Children's Tylenol (160mg/5mL) every 4-6 hours.

The most common responsible viruses for the blisters (ulcers) in the mouth are Entroviruses. Enterovirus 71 is associated with Hand-Foot and Mouth disease and Herpangina. Benadryl elixir and Maalox regular strength, a ½ teaspoon of the mix given in a 1:1 ratio, can also be used to coat the ulcers and sooth the mouth.

## CASE #110

MID-SPRING

A three-year-old female child

CC: Head trauma & laceration

The foster mother states that the child fell in the park and hit her head on the ground. She denies a loss of consciousness, but she states that the child has an open cut on the back of her head. An ice pack was applied.

Disposition: The foster mother is advised to take the child to the ED to be examined and to have the wound closed. Her immunization record should be checked, and if she is not up to date for DTaP immunization, then she should receive a Tetanus or DTaP immunization.

## Case #111

Time: 11:00PM

A six-year-old male child

CC: Asthma & allergy problem; question about the medicine
The child has a history of asthma and an allergic rhinitis problem. His mother had a question regarding the allergy medication, Benadryl.
Disposition: If the child is on Benadryl for his allergies, then he should be drinking more fluid to be well-hydrated, so that dryness and thickening of the nasal secretions can be prevented. The mother is also advised to keep the child's appointment for his asthma follow-up.

## Case #112

Mid-spring Time: 10:15PM

A one-year-old male infant

CC: Rash
The infant had received his one-year-old immunizations last week and has developed a rash. The mother is advised that one of the immunizations he had received at one year of age was the MMR.
Disposition: The mother is advised that sometimes in one week to ten days after the MMR immunization, children may develop a rash that is similar to the rash in mild measles disease and that the rash will improve after a few days. She is instructed to observe the infant, and keep his appointments as scheduled.

## Case #113

Mid-spring Time: 11:35PM

A two-year-old male toddler

CC: Complaining after using ear drops
The child had Tympanostomy tubes placed in his ears recently. He complains about his

left ear. He was seen by an ENT physician and is on Sulfacetamide ear drops. The ear drops were just started but the toddler cannot tolerate them, and he complains with each application.

Disposition: His mother is advised to hold the bottle of ear drops in the palms of her hands to make the liquid warmer, prior to using them. She is to continue to use the drops as instructed and to watch for any reaction to the medicine. She may contact the specialist in the morning, to see if a change in medication is advised.

## CASE #114
LATE WINTER                                                    TIME: 5:50PM

A ten-month-old male infant

CC: Fever & a history of bronchiolitis

The infant has had a fever, with a temperature 101.3°F (38.5°C) today. His mother states that the infant has a new fever but has been having a cough since about six or seven days ago. He was seen at the hospital and she was told the infant had Bronchiolitis.

Disposition: The mother is advised to give the infant Tylenol (Infants' Tylenol every 4-6 hours for fever) and fluid (juice, broth) and observe. If the infant continues having fevers, then he is to be reexamined in the morning. The timing of the fever is worrisome for a potential secondary infection, like an ear infection. However, the height of the fever is low, and the child can wait to be rechecked in the morning if not in any respiratory distress.

## CASE #115
LATE WINTER                                                    TIME: 5:55PM

A seven-week-old female neonate

CC: Facial rash

The mother states that the baby has a rash on her face. The mother has been using soap on the neonate's face.

Disposition: The mother is advised that she should avoid using soap on the baby's face to prevent irritation of the face and to observe. Excessive washing and soaps can be drying to the baby's sensitive skin. The baby can be checked at the clinic if required.

## Case #116

TIME: 6:08PM

An eight-year-old female child

CC: Myasthenia gravis & medication refill request
Her mother states that the child has Myasthenia gravis and is on Mestinon Syrup. She has run out of the medication.
Disposition: The prescription Mestinon (Pyridostigmine Bromide) is ordered directly to the pharmacy and is to be picked up by the child's parents. The mother is also advised to please keep the child's appointment for follow-up.

## Case #117

LATE WINTER                                                 TIME: 7:46PM

A two-month-old male infant

CC: Constipation
His mother states that the infant is constipated and she denies any other problem. The baby has been pushing to defecate and his stool is hard and there is only a small amount of stool. The bowel movements are not daily.
Disposition: The mother is advised to offer the baby some water to drink (4oz.) and to observe. The infant is to be examined if the constipation persists or if child vomits or is cranky. She may try small amounts (one tablespoon) of juice like prune or pear juice and observe, or alternatively an ounce of one of these juices may be diluted with 4oz. of water. She can also bicycle the baby's legs, massage the belly in a clockwise fashion, and gently take a rectal temperature, using a little bit of Vaseline to the tip of the rectal thermometer.

## Case #118

LATE WINTER                                                 TIME: 9:29PM

A one-year-old male infant

CC: Slight fever & one episode of vomiting
The mother states that the infant has a slight fever and has vomited once today. The child was seen by his pediatrician yesterday and received his immunizations: MMR, Varicella vaccine, Prevnar (Strep Pneumoniae), Comvax (Hepatitis B and Hemophilus

influenza type B vaccine).

Disposition: The mother is advised to give the baby Infants' Tylenol every 4-6 hours for fever (temperature ≥100.4°F [38.0°C]) and offer him more fluid (Juice, water, Pedialyte) and to observe. The baby may be checked if the condition persists.

A slight fever after some immunizations are expected, but the infant should be observed to see if he is developing a viral infection or another condition.

## CASE #119

An eight-month-old female infant

CC: Rash following taking Amoxicillin

The father states that the infant had an ear infection six days ago. She was seen by the pediatrician and received Amoxicillin, but the child has now developed a rash. The parents have stopped the antibiotics.

Disposition: The father is advised to observe the child and if she is symptomatic and develops any fever, then she is to be reexamined. The infant should have a follow-up appointment. They can also try a dose of Benadryl to see if the rash is ameliorated with that measure.

## CASE #120

A 19-month-old female toddler

CC: Pink eye

The mother states the child has pink eyes.

Disposition: She is advised to clean the eyes with cool sterile water and make an appointment for today to be examined.

The responsible virus usually is adenovirus with no seasonality prevalence. Other agents including bacteria should be considered, especially if discharge is noted or if there is eyelash mattering.

## CASE #121

A one-year-old female infant

CC: Fever

The infant has a fever, she was seen at the ED and acetaminophen syrup was advised. The child has had no vomiting and has been drinking well.

Disposition: The mother is advised regarding giving acetaminophen (every 4-6 hours) for a temperature ≥100.4°F (38.0°C), to offer her enough fluid (juice, water) and to observe. In case the condition persists, and there is a fever ≥102.2°F-102.5°F (39.0-39.1°C), then the infant may be reexamined.


## Case #122

Early summer                                                    Time: 10:02AM

A four-month-old male infant

CC: Cough & cold

The mother states that the infant has been having cough and cold symptoms for three days. He has also been having a fever, with a temperature of 101.0°F (38.3°C) for three days, and greenish mucus from his nose.

Disposition: The mother is advised to have the infant checked given his young age and respiratory symptoms. The mother is also advised to use Normal Saline nose drops in his nostrils (one to two drops three or four times per day) and Infants' Tylenol (every four to six hours) are to be given for fever. An infant with greenish mucus and fever should be checked.


## Case #123

Early summer                                                    Time: 11:30AM

An 18-year-old female adolescent

CC: Adolescent with cough, fever, & pregnancy

The teen states that she has cough and fever and likewise that she is pregnant. She thinks she has pneumonia.

Disposition: She is advised to be checked. She is also advised that she should be well-hydrated and she should be drinking extra fluid (water, juice and soup) to alleviate her cough, and that she should continue to take her prenatal vitamins.


## Case #124

Early summer                                                    Time: 12:18PM

A 17-month-old male toddler

CC: Cold symptoms
The mother states the child has cold symptoms and that he has no fever.
Disposition: The mother is advised to use Normal Saline nose drops in the child's nostrils (one or two drops a few times per day), to offer him more fluid (juice, soup, ginger ale) to drink, and to observe. Have the toddler checked if required (if refusing to drink, not voiding, or if worsening).

## CASE #125
EARLY SUMMER                                          TIME: 12:27PM

A two-month-old male infant

CC: Intermittent crying
The father states that the infant cries sometimes, he has neither fever nor vomiting. He has had a normal bowel movement last night. He is breastfeeding well.
Disposition: The father is advised that as the infant may have no other problems, occasional crying could be normal. The infant should be cuddled and swaddled. The father should make sure that the infant's clothing is comfortable and he is not wet nor hungry. The infant is to be observed. The infant is to be examined if required. Reflux precautions like holding the baby upright after each feeding, elevating the head of the crib, giving smaller more frequent feedings and burping more frequently may also help. Sometimes the crying is related to the colic. Recently colic has been associated with a lack of good bacteria in the child's intestines and so the use of probiotics is advised. That was not the case in the past. Alternatively, depending on the mother's diet, sometimes there may be a component of the maternal breastmilk that may be causing more gas. The mother could try to avoid drinking cow's milk and gas-producing foods like beans, onion, cauliflower and radishes and see if there is a difference. If the crying worsens and the baby is very fussy and hard to console, then the baby must be checked.

## CASE #126
EARLY SUMMER                                          TIME: 1:10PM

A two-month-old female infant

CC: Rash
The mother states that the infant has a pinpoint rash all over the body especially

around her neck. She has no fever, no vomiting and no other problem. She is not fussy and is feeding and voiding normally.

Disposition: The mother is advised regarding the heat rash, she is to avoid over-dressing the baby, to bathe her more often and is to use cornstarch powder (not talc) around her neck (by gently placing some there with her hand, not by pouring the powder [to prevent inhalation of the powder]) and to then observe. Clothes and blankets should be 100% cotton. If the infant has any additional problems, then she can be checked today.

## CASE #127
EARLY SUMMER                                                    TIME: 2:25PM

A five-year-old female child

CC: Earache
Her mother states that the child complains of an earache. Tylenol was given but she still complains of pain despite the pain medication.

Disposition: The mother is advised to take the child to be checked. An earache is often associated with an infection. The child may be checked in the daytime and receive antibiotic if required.

## CASE #128
EARLY SUMMER                                                    TIME: 3:30PM

A three-month-old male infant

CC: Sore in the mouth
His mother states that the infant has a sore in his mouth. He is breastfeeding and the mother also has sore nipples.

Disposition: The mother is advised regarding the oral hygiene of the infant, and to offer him small amount of cool boiled water after the feedings to wash out the mouth. The mother is to take care of her own nipples and express her milk to give to the infant. The infant may be checked tomorrow if required (if the sores persist, or if the feedings are not going as well as they had been).

## CASE #129
EARLY SUMMER                                                    TIME: 4:20PM

A nine-month-old male infant

CC: Bleeding from the site of tube insertion in the eardrum

His mother states that the infant has an ear problem. He just had a Tympanostomy tube inserted to his eardrum and now has had some bleeding.

Disposition: The mother is advised that if the bleeding has currently stopped, and there is just a drop or two of blood, that it may be acceptable and that he will be fine. She should just clean the blood in the outside of the ear and observe. However, if there is active bleeding, then it is better to have the infant checked.

## CASE #130

EARLY SUMMER                                                      TIME: 11:00PM

A nine-month-old male infant

CC: Cough & vomiting after the cough

The infant has a cough and sometimes vomits after the cough.

Disposition: His father is advised regarding feeding him smaller amounts but in shorter intervals to prevent vomiting after the cough, making sure the infant has no wheezing (noisy breathing) and making sure that he is not in any distress. He may be checked tomorrow if these conditions are met. Most infections with enterovirus occur in the summer and fall; some are associated with respiratory manifestations.

## CASE #131

EARLY SUMMER                                                      TIME: 11:20PM

A six-week-old male neonate

CC: Vomiting forcefully

His mother states that the baby had vomiting a few days ago. He was hospitalized for one or two days. He was then discharged and the parents have been told he is fine. Now he vomited once rather forcefully.

Disposition: The mother is advised to offer him small amounts of Pedialyte and to observe. The baby should be reevaluated if he continues to vomit. Ruling out pyloric stenosis should be kept in mind.

## CASE #132

EARLY SUMMER                                                      TIME: 8:00PM

A two-year-old-female toddler

CC: Fever

Her mother states that the child has developed a fever today. She had a temperature of 101.6°F (38.6°C) and received Tylenol. Her temperature is coming back again.

Disposition: Her mother is advised regarding giving Tylenol syrup 160mg/5mL every four to six hours for temperature ≥ 100.4°F (38.0°C), offering her fluid (water, juice and soup), and observing. If the fever persists, and is ≥102.2-102.5°F (39.0-39.1°C) then the toddler may be checked at the ED. Otherwise, she can be checked at the doctor's office or clinic the following day for lower temperatures, should the mother want.

## CASE #133

EARLY SUMMER                                                    TIME: 7:40PM

A 19-year-old female adolescent

CC: Vaginal bleeding & possible pregnancy

The adolescent has vaginal bleeding and her mother thinks she is pregnant.

Disposition: Her mother is advised to take her to the gynecologist. If she is in any distress (looks weak, pale and loosing blood), she should be seen at the ED. An adolescent with vaginal bleeding who could potentially be pregnancy should be evaluated for ectopic pregnancy, ruptures, and placenta previa.

## CASE #134

MID-WINTER                                                     TIME: 4:08PM

A ten-month-old male infant

CC: Bleeding from the prepuce

His mother is anxious because while she was retracting the prepuce, the infant had some bleeding.

Disposition: The mother is advised to keep the bleeding area clean. She may use a tear-free baby shampoo to clean the prepuce. Avoid retracting the prepuce. She may apply Bacitracin ointment on the area 3 times per day for a few days.

## CASE #135

MID-WINTER                                                     TIME: 5:00PM

A two-year-old male toddler

CC: Cough & asthma

The child is an asthmatic and has been coughing. He is on Pulmicort and Xopenex via the nebulizer. There is no respiratory distress (no fast breathing, no nasal flaring or retractions, nor abdominal breathing).

Disposition: The mother is advised to use his medications as instructed, keep him well-hydrated, and to observe.

Pulmicort Respules (Budesonide in micronized form 0.25mg/2mL suspension for inhalation) relieves the swelling of the airways.

Xopenex (beta 2 agonists, levalbuterol, as HCL, single-isomer albuterol, 0.31mg/3mL inhalation solution) relaxes the muscles of the airways. Both medications help to open-up the airways and help the child breathe better. The mother also is advised to keep the appointment for his asthma follow-up as scheduled.

## CASE #136

MID-WINTER                                                TIME: 5:30PM

A nine-month-old female infant

CC: Vomiting

The infant has vomited once today and she also vomited once last night. There was neither blood nor bile in the vomit.

She has neither fever nor any other problem. She has not had any bowel movement today, and she had normal bowel movements yesterday.

Disposition: Her mother is advised to keep the infant on clear fluid like Pedialyte and to observe. If she cannot retain the Pedialyte, then she should have her examined at the ED. During the winter, influenza and other respiratory virus infections may be responsible for gastroenteritis symptoms. Rotavirus infection is also more common during the cool seasons.

## CASE #137

MID-WINTER                                                TIME: 7:00PM

A 13-year-old male adolescent

CC: Dizziness & fainting

The adolescent had an episode of dizziness and fainting in school, while he was standing yesterday. He was checked by the school nurse, and has been told he was okay. He has no current symptoms.

Disposition: The mother is advised to make sure he eats properly before going to school, that he is well-hydrated, and to observe. If he has any complaints, then he can be checked tonight at the ED (it is the weekend). Otherwise, he may have a complete check-up on Monday at the clinic. His blood pressure (lying, sitting and standing), fasting blood sugar, a complete blood count, and an electrocardiogram (ECG) may be among the primary studies to be done for fainting.

## Case #138

Mid-winter                                                                Time: 8:15PM

A four-year-old female child

CC: Fever & sore throat

The child has been having a fever and sore throat since yesterday. Her temperature is 102.0°F (38.8°C) now; Tylenol (160mg/5mL) has been given to her. She has not had any vomiting. She has been coughing. Her mother has been giving her Robitussin Cough syrup.

Disposition: The mother is advised to continue to give her Tylenol syrup 160mg/5mL every four to six hours for temperature ≥100.4°F (38.0°C), to offer her more fluid (juice, soup, water) and to observe. Motrin can also be offered. If she continues having a high fever despite Tylenol and Motrin, then she is to be examined at the ED. However, if the fever responds to the antipyretics (Tylenol and Motrin) then she can be seen in clinic the next day.

Over-the-counter cough syrup and cold medications are no longer advised for the children under age 6 years. Taking extra fluids moisturizes the mucous membranes of respiratory tracts and so acts as an expectorant. Use of a humidifier is also helpful. A child with a persistent fever that is not coming down easily with antipyretics might be showing a sign of having a bacterial infection, and so can be checked sooner.

## Case #139

Mid-winter                                                                Time: 4:00PM

A six-year-old male child

CC: Dysuria

His mother states that the child complains of a burning sensation when he urinates, and that this started this afternoon. He denies any trauma to that area. He is not circumcised. His mother noticed mild redness to the penis tip with blood crust in the prepuce area.

Disposition: The mother is advised to use Bacitracin ointment on that area (prepuce and the tip of his penis) and to have the child checked tomorrow.

## CASE #140
MID-WINTER                                                                    TIME: 4:47PM

A four-month-old male infant

CC: Runny nose & slight fever

His mother states that the infant started to have a runny nose and temperature 99-101.0°F (37.2-38.3°C) today. He is a little cranky.

Disposition: The mother is advised to give him Infants' Tylenol for fever, to use Normal Saline nose drops (1-2 drops in his nostrils, 3-4 times per day), and to observe. The viral pathogens responsible for cold symptoms include rhinoviruses, adenoviruses, influenza viruses, parainfluenza viruses and respiratory syncytial virus (RSV). Sometimes viral respiratory infection is associated with a secondary bacterial infection. If the temperature persists or the infant's temperature is ≥102.2°F (39.0°C), then the infant should be checked sooner.

## CASE #141
MID-WINTER                                                                    TIME: 6:34PM

A five-year-old male preschooler

CC: Vomiting

The child has been vomiting. He vomited once last night, and once today. There is no blood nor bile in the vomit. He also complains of abdominal pain off and on since yesterday. He had a normal bowel movement yesterday, and has not had any bowel movement today. He had some rice and beans today.

Disposition: His mother is advised to give him just clear fluid (Pedialyte, Gatorade, ginger ale, water) for a couple hours and to observe. If his pain increases or the vomiting persists, and he cannot keep down the clear liquids, then he is to be examined.

## CASE #142
MID-WINTER                                                                    TIME: 7:00PM

A five-year-old female preschooler

CC: Vulvar itch & whitish vaginal discharge after recent prolonged antibiotic use

The child has had a recent history of an ear infection two weeks ago and has been on the antibiotic Augmentin for almost two weeks. She now has itching in her vaginal area with a whitish discharge. Her mother has Clotrimazole 1% cream at home.

Disposition: The mother is advised to use the Clotrimazole cream on the vulva (the itchy area, externally) twice per day and to observe. If she is not improving, she may be checked tomorrow at the clinic. Prolonged use of antibiotic causes an increased susceptibility to fungal infection.

## Case #143

Mid-winter                                                                Time: 7:35 PM

A three-week-old female neonate

CC: Spitting-up frequently

The infant has been spitting-up frequently. She was seen by her pediatrician today, and was told that she has been gaining weight properly. The mother wants to change to a soy-based formula.

Disposition: The mother is advised to avoid over feeding the baby, and to have a good feeding technique. She also is advised to keep the infant in upright position for about 20 minutes after each feeding. At this point, there is no need to change the formula, but, if she would like, she may change the formula to soy-based formula (the neonate was born full term) and observe. The baby may be reexamined if the condition persists.

## Case #144

Mid-winter                                                                Time: 8:37PM

A one-year-old female infant

CC: A chief complaint was not mentioned; the mother was just wanting a callback.

Unfortunately, the telephone number given to the answering service was not correct. Thus, I could not get in-touch with the family. The answering service was advised to wait and see if the caregiver calls back.

Difficulty reaching the family is also a part of the on-call experience.

## Case #145

Mid-winter                                                                Time: 10:34PM

A three-year-old male child with special needs

CC: Cough & choking on his phlegm, diarrhea
The child has had a cough and has been choking on his phlegm. He has also diarrhea tonight.
Disposition: His mother is advised to give him clear fluid (Pedialyte, water, Gatorade) and to keep his airway open by using Normal Saline nose drops (1-2 drops, three or four times per day) in his nostrils, and to use a humidifier around him. If there is any distress, then he will need to be seen at the hospital tonight.


## Case #147

Mid-winter                                             Time: 11:51PM

A ten-year-old female child

CC: Fever & nausea
The father states that the child has a fever and nausea tonight. Her temperature, taken via an ear probe device, is 103.4°F (39.6°C).
Disposition: The father is advised to give her Motrin 100mg/5mL, to offer her fluid, and to recheck the temperature. If she is not having a good response to these interventions, then she can be examined at the ED tonight. However, if the temperature is coming down and her condition is good, then it is best that she be checked tomorrow morning. The father should give her Motrin every 6-8 hours for a temperature ≥100.4°F (38.0°C). When the temperature persists (is unchanged) despite antipyretics, this can be a sign of having a bacterial infection and so the child can be checked sooner, rather than later.


## Case #147

Mid-winter                                             Time: 12:33AM

A one-month-old male neonate

CC: Nasal congestion
The neonate has been having nasal congestion since shortly after birth. He is feeding well, voiding well, acting normally and has had no fever.
Disposition: The mother is advised to use Normal Saline nose drops (one or two drops into the nostrils, three or four times per day), to use a humidifier in the room, and to observe.

# Case #148

A one-month-old female neonate

CC: Cough
The neonate has been having a cough for three to four days.
Disposition: The mother is advised that if the child has no fever, and is not in any distress, then Normal Saline nose drops and a humidifier can be used and the infant may be checked in the walk-in clinic later today. Otherwise, if she is in any distress (coughing a great deal, having rapid breathing, nasal flaring, or retractions) then she can call 911 or take the baby to the ED. If she were to have a fever (rectal temperature ≥100.4°F [38.0°C]), then she should be checked at the ED, given the young age.

# Case #149

Early autumn                                    Time: 4:40PM

A nine-day-old male neonate

CC: Umbilical stump partially wet
His mother states the baby's umbilical cord fell off yesterday but that a part of the umbilical stump is still wet.
Disposition: The mother is advised to clean the umbilical stump with rubbing alcohol and to observe. If there is any discharge, or foul odor from the umbilical stump, or any redness around the umbilical area, then the neonate is to be examined tonight. Otherwise, he can be checked in clinic the next day. When there are, bacteria colonized on the umbilical stump, it can cause omphalitis. It should be diagnosed early and treated to prevent serious complications.

# Case #150

Early autumn                                    Time: 4:50PM

A three-year-old female child

CC: Insect bite
Her mother states that the child had one itchy bump on her leg yesterday. Her mother rubbed alcohol on it, and it appears better today, but she has two or three more bumps on her leg and they are itchy.

Disposition: Her mother is advised to use Calamine lotion on the bumps and try to prevent insect bites. She should also have her wear long sleeves and long pants, use an insect repellent, and observe. If the child complains of pain, or has any redness or warmth at the site of the insect bites, then the child may be checked at that point.

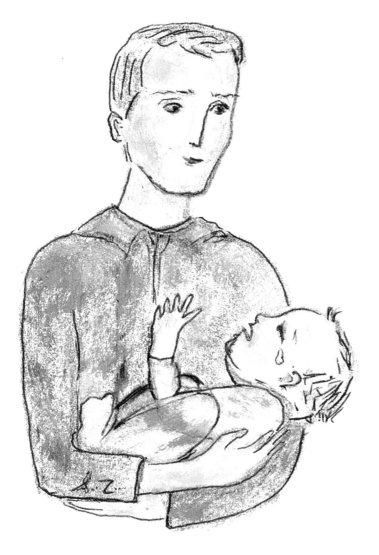

Case #125

A 2-month-old infant with crying

# Chapter Four

---

## Case #151

Early autumn                                                    Time: 7:03PM

A six-week-old male neonate

CC: Colic & a rash to the back of the ears

His mother states that the infant has colic and has a rash behind his ears. He is feeding well and voiding well. There has been neither vomiting nor spit-up. The baby is just crying a bit more than is usual for him, and has a rash that she has just noticed.

Disposition: The mother is advised on how to alleviate the colic by cuddling/swaddling the baby at the time of crying. The mother is also advised on reflux precautions (holding the baby vertically for 20 minutes after each feeding, elevating the head of the crib, burping the child more frequently and giving smaller amounts more frequently). She should make sure not to overfeed him and observe. If the baby can be consoled with these measures, there is no urgency in getting him checked tonight. If she cannot console the baby, then he can be seen in the ED.

The rash to the back of his ears could be seborrhea, also known as seborrheic dermatitis. She may use a moisturizing lotion like Aquaphor or Cetaphil as well as mild steroid cream like hydrocortisone 1% to see if it helps the rash. Also, a baby shampoo or an anti-seborrheic shampoo like Selenium sulfide, Sulfur or tar shampoo, may be used once a week. Mother is advised to make an appointment for the baby to be checked at the clinic.

## Case #152

Early autumn                                                    Time: 9:17PM

A one-month-old male neonate

CC: Fever
The infant has a fever; his temperature has been 101.0°F (38.3°C) since last night.
Disposition: His mother is advised to take the infant to the emergency department (ED) right away.
A neonate with a fever should be checked immediately when the fever is noticed, as these infants are most at risk for serious bacterial infections including meningitis, bacteremia (blood infections) and urinary tract infections.

## Case #153
Early autumn                                          Time: 10:15PM

A three-week-old male neonate

CC: Constipation
The neonate has not had any bowel movements for two days. He takes both breastmilk and Similac with iron formula. He usually had been having three or four bowel movements per day. He has had no vomiting. He is not cranky. His abdomen is soft according to his mother.
Disposition: The mother is advised to massage the abdomen, to try to increase the amount of breastmilk offered, and to bicycle the baby's legs. She can also gently take a rectal temperature, using a little Vaseline. She may also offer the baby some water (cool boiled water) to drink (just 2-4oz.) and should please keep the appointment to be examined tomorrow.

## Case #154
Mid-summer                                            Time: 6:44PM

A ten-month-old male infant

CC: Crankiness
The infant has been crying off-and-on since about 10:00PM last night. The infant had a cough and cold the prior week. He was seen at a clinic and received an antibiotic which has not been properly administered. He was seen by a physician two days ago, because of fever, and the use of Tylenol was advised. His bowel movements are normal.
Disposition: The mother is advised to have the baby reexamined today. It is possible that the antibiotics were for an ear infection and, as there was poor compliance with

the medication, the infection may be still being present and may be causing the baby pain.

## CASE #155

A 13-month-old female infant

CC: Diarrhea

The child had diarrhea and fever three or four days ago, the mother was called by the nurse and was told that the child needs an antibiotic because of an intestinal infection. She was told that the physician will call and prescribe antibiotics for the baby. She has not heard from her doctor yet. The child has no fever now. She had two normal bowel movements, with no blood and no mucus in the stool.

Disposition: The mother is advised to please call tomorrow morning and inquire regarding the stool test result and the antibiotic.

As this was a time before the advent of the electronic medical record, I could not access the records of a colleague, and so had no way to follow-up on the lab results and physician plan. As the infant was not having bloody stools and was in good condition, it was okay to wait until the following day, to have the mother speak to the infant's physician directly.

## CASE #156

A two-year-old male toddler

CC: Fever

The child has been having a fever since last night. He has had no vomiting. Tylenol was given, and the temperature had come down, but he is developing a fever again as it is wearing off. His bowel movements are normal. His appetite is less than usual.

Disposition: The mother is advised to give him Children's Tylenol (160mg/5mL) every 4-6 hours for a temperature ≥100.4°F (38.0°C), and to offer him more fluid (water, juice, soup, ginger ale) to drink. Children's Motrin can also be given. If his temperature goes above 102.2°F (39.0°C), then he can be checked tomorrow morning. If the temperature is not coming down with Tylenol and Motrin, or if he develops more symptoms that worry the mother, he can be checked sooner if need be.

## Case #157

Time: 7:43PM

A three-month-old female infant

CC: Moving a great deal

The mother states that the baby had his 2-month immunizations 16 days ago. She has been fine but she appears to be irritable for the past two days. She has had no fever, no excessive crying, no vomiting, and no diarrhea, but appears to be moving a great deal. Disposition: The mother is advised if the infant is otherwise fine, then she can wait and call tomorrow morning to have the baby examined. The movement of the three-month-old infant could be normal but should be observed by a physician, and the immunization history may be reviewed. The complaints do not appear to be related to the immunizations.

## Case #158

Mid-summer                                                              Time: 12:25AM

A nine-month-old female infant

CC: Fever & crankiness

The infant has a fever, with a temperature of 103.1°F (39.5°C). She was seen by a physician at the ED two days ago, and the mother was told that she had an ear infection. She has been on Motrin and Amoxicillin since then. However, she continues to have a fever, and has been cranky and vomits sometimes.
Disposition: The mother is advised to take the baby to the ED to be reevaluated, as the Motrin is not helping neither the fever nor crankiness. The infant might have a viral infection or the ear infection might not be responding to the Amoxicillin. Her ears should be rechecked and a decision made accordingly. Perhaps it will be necessary that further work-up be done. A child on antibiotics should not continue to have high fevers after 48-72 hours on the appropriate medication, if she is indeed responding to the medicine.

## Case #159

Mid-summer                                                              Time: 4:50PM

A 14-day-old male neonate

CC: Listlessness

His foster mother states that the infant has been very quiet today. He is not drinking his formula properly. The foster mother states that the baby has a soft cleft palate and that he has been vomiting frequently in the last six days, which is when the foster mother had first received him. He also has a history of maternal drug abuse. The infant had an abdominal sonogram yesterday.

Disposition: The foster mother is advised to take the neonate to the ED for an evaluation, she may call 911. The neonate is listless and perhaps is dehydrated because of feeding difficulty and vomiting.

## CASE #160

MID-SUMMER                                                    TIME: 7:30PM

An eleven-month-old male infant

CC: Blisters on toes due to the new large sneakers

His mother states she just has purchased a pair of sneakers for the infant. They appear to be too large for him and due to his skin rubbing against the sneakers while he walks, he has developed blisters on his small toes on both feet.

Disposition: The mother is advised to keep the feet clean, obtain an antibiotic ointment, like Bacitracin ointment, and then apply it over the affected area three times per day for five to seven days, and observe. If there is any fever, redness, etc. then she may have the infant examined. Avoid shoes for now, and in the future, please make sure the shoes fit well.

## CASE #161

MID-SUMMER                                                    TIME: 8:00PM

A three-week-old female neonate

CC: Rash

The baby has a fine rash over her forehead, cheeks and neck. She is fine otherwise. She takes her formula well, and is not cranky. There is no history of maternal infection, and she had no problems after birth.

Disposition: The mother is advised to avoid over warming the baby, and thus prevent sweating. She also is advised that she should bathe the baby, and use cornstarch powder (not talc) around her neck (after placing it on her hand first, to avoid inhalation) and to observe. If the rash is not getting better or if there is any other problem, then she may have the baby checked.

# Case #162

A six-month-old female infant

CC: Fever & rash after taking Tylenol

The infant has a fever; her temperature is 101.0°F (38.3°C) today.

Her temperature was not taken yesterday. She has had no vomiting. She was checked by her Pediatrician today. She was told that her throat was slightly congested, and Tylenol was advised. She has developed patches of rash on her face, and on the back of her neck, after taking the Tylenol.

Disposition: The mother is advised not to give her Tylenol. For the fever, she can give her Children's Motrin 100mg/5mL, for true fever (temperature ≥100.4°F [38.0°C]), every 6 to 8 hours, and she may use Calamine lotion on the rash if it appears to be bothersome for the infant, and observe. The infant may be reexamined if the fever persists or if another problem arises.

# Case #163

Mid-summer                                                           Time: 11:11PM

A 15-month-old female toddler

CC: Fever & rash

The toddler has had a fever, temperature of 101.7°F (38.7°C) today. She also had a slight fever yesterday. She has had no vomiting. She has red spots on her face and body. She received Motrin about a half an hour ago.

Disposition: The mother is advised that if the fever responds to Motrin and comes down, then she can wait until tomorrow to be seen. Otherwise, she should take the child to the ED to be examined tonight if the fever were to get above 102.5°F (39.1°C). Most enterovirus infections occur in summer and fall.

# Case #164

Mid -summer                                                          Time: 4:58AM

A four-month-old female infant

CC: Cough & spitting up mucus

The infant has been coughing a great deal and spiting-up mucus. He has neither fever nor vomiting. He refuses to take formula, and has been taking only juice for the past two days.

Disposition: The mother is advised to take the infant to the ED to be examined. Since the infant has been on only juice for 2 days, the electrolytes may be imbalanced. She should have been given a fluid containing electrolytes (Pedialyte) to prevent hyponatremia (low blood sodium). Also, he has been coughing a great deal and is very young, so it is better that he be checked.

## Case #165

Mid-summer                                                                Time: 7:50AM

A 12-day-old female neonate

CC: Thrush & vomiting the medicine

The neonate has been vomiting five to ten minutes after having taken 2 mL of the medicine, Nystatin oral suspension, for the treatment of the oral thrush. Her mother states that the baby was seen by her pediatrician yesterday and is on 2mL of Nystatin 4 times per day.

Disposition: The mother is advised to reduce the dose of Nystatin to one mL, four times per day, and to observe.

One to two milliliters of Nystatin (Mycostatin, Nilstat) oral suspension, four times per day, is used on the whitish spots and the baby then swallows the medicine. This usually works for the treatment of oral Thrush. Each mL of Nystatin oral suspension contains 100,000 units. Alternatively, she can paint the tongue, inside of the mouth, gums with Nystatin, and she may use a Q-tip to do so if this is easier for her. Once the spots are gone, the medicine should be used for an additional 3 days, as the thrush is usually still present on a microscopic level.

## Case #166

Mid-summer                                                                Time: 8:35AM

A 20-month-old female infant

CC: Diarrhea & vomiting

The toddler had been having a fever for two days. She was seen by her Pediatrician, and received Amoxicillin 250mg/5mL oral suspension to be given three times per day for an early ear infection. The child has no fever today, but now has vomiting and diarrhea. She has been having loose bowel movements three times today.

Disposition: The mother is advised to offer Pedialyte to the child for 12 to 24 hours and to observe. If she cannot retain the Pedialyte, she may be examined at the ED. If the vomiting improves, then in addition to giving her Pedialyte and clear fluids (white grape juice and ginger ale), she is to offer her foods like white rice, applesauce, saltine or graham crackers, banana and plain yogurt. The toddler should have a follow-up appointment to be checked if she is not improving.

## Case #167

A nine-month-old male infant

CC: Rash

A rash was noticed today on the baby's face, trunk and his extremities. His mother states that the infant has had a cold for a while and has been teething. He was seen by his pediatrician eleven days ago. He was put on albuterol syrup 2.5mL every 8 hours for the cough, and it was just given once. The infant has had a facial rash for a few days. His mother gave him strawberries yesterday for the first time. He has had neither fever nor vomiting. There is no breathing difficulty.

Disposition: The mother is advised to avoid giving the infant hyper-allergenic foods (eggs, strawberries, tomato sauce, and seafood) and to use calamine lotion on the rash. If his cough persists, then she may continue the albuterol syrup for this as was instructed and observe. If the condition persists or the rash is not resolving, then the baby may be checked.

## Case #168

Mid-summer                                                                    Time: 2:05AM

An 18-month-old male infant

CC: Fever

The child has a fever; her temp is 103.6°F (39.7°C) now. About one hour ago, his temperature was 103.2°F (39.5°C) and Motrin was given. His father states that the infant started to have a fever yesterday afternoon, and that he also has been having a slight cough. He also vomited once after taking the Motrin, and he has a history of previous ear infections.

Disposition: The father is advised to take the child to the ED.

An eighteen-month old toddler with high fever (temperature ≥102.2-102.5°F

[39.0-39.1ºC]) should be checked, as there may be a bacterial source for the fevers. Infants and toddlers are more at risk for these infections given their younger age (<3 years old).

## CASE #169

MID-SUMMER                                                    TIME: 12:30PM

A two-year-old male toddler

CC: Sore to the corner of lips
The child has a sore to the corner of his lips for about 4-5 days. He has history of viral infection of the mouth a while ago which improved.
Disposition: The mother is advised to offer him mild and soft foods and nothing that would irritate his mouth. She is to give him multivitamin drops (one mL daily) and to rinse his mouth with cool water after he eats. She may also use a little Bacitracin ointment on the sore at the corner of the lips three times per day, and observe. The toddler is to be examined if the condition persists. Enterovirus infections occur in the summer time. They have variable clinical manifestations. Herpangina, stomatitis and Hand, Foot and Mouth Disease are some common enteroviral infections. Vitamin deficiency is one of the factors that cause perleche (sores to the corner of the mouth).

## CASE #170

MID-SUMMER                                                    TIME: 7:50PM

A 16-month-old male infant

CC: Fever, medication question about the dose of Infants' Tylenol
The infant has a temperature of 101.0ºF (38.3ºC). His mother would like to know how much Tylenol she can give the infant. The child has a slight cough and has been sneezing.
Disposition: The dose is calculated for the mother based on the toddler's weight and so the mother is advised to give him 80mg of Infants' Tylenol every four hours for temperatures ≥100.4ºF (38.0ºC), and to offer him more fluids (water, juice, soup) to drink when he has a fever, and to observe. If the fevers are ≥102.2ºF (39.0ºC), the child can be given an appointment at that time.

## Case #171

A five-month-old male infant

CC: Cold, cough & sneezing
The infant has had cold symptoms since yesterday with coughing and sneezing. He vomited once last night after feeding. His temperature is 102.0°F (38.8°C) today. Tylenol was given and he is sleeping now.
Disposition: The mother is advised to recheck the temperature later. If the infant continues to have a fever, and the fever is higher than 102.2°F (39.0°C), then the infant may be examined today. It is best to examine a five-month-old infant with a high fever.

## Case #172

Mid-summer          Time: 9:38AM

An 18-month-old male toddler

CC: Earache
The mother states that the child appears to have left earache. He has neither a fever nor cold symptoms. The mother just gave him one teaspoon of Children's Motrin syrup.
Disposition: The mother is advised that if the child is not complaining, and is fine with the Motrin, then she may wait until tomorrow to have the toddler checked at the clinic. Otherwise, if she cannot control his pain then she may take him to the ED to be examined today (weekend call).

## Case #173

Mid-summer          Time: 2:46PM

A twelve-month-old female infant

CC: Baby dislikes regular cow's milk, prefers formula
The mother states the child is one-year-old and she just started the cow's milk for her. The child does not like the regular cow's milk and likes the formula Enfamil with iron.
Disposition: The mother is advised that she may continue the formula and gradually introduce the cow's milk to the infant's diet, and to keep her appointment at the pediatric clinic as already scheduled.

## Case #174

A 16-month-old female toddler

CC: Insect bite

The child has multiple mosquito bites on her exposed areas like her face and extremities. She has no fever. The mother states that the child had the same problem a few months ago, and was told that she had the chickenpox. There is no sign of skin infection around the lesions, like redness or swelling on the site of the lesions.

Disposition: The mother is advised to apply Calamine lotion on the skin lesions, and to observe. If she wants to be checked in the morning, she may call tomorrow to be checked at the clinic (weekend call).

## Case #175

Mid-summer

Time: 4:37PM

A ten-month-old male infant

CC: Fever

The infant has had a fever. He has been having a fever for two days. His temperature is 101.7°F (38.7°C) and Tylenol was given about 2 hours ago. The mother states that the baby is teething and that he looks well. He has had no vomiting, nor has he had any mucus from his nose. He has been drinking well.

Disposition: The mother is advised to give him Children's Motrin syrup (100mg/5mL) and to observe. If the fever comes down, she may wait until tomorrow to have the baby checked should she desire. An infant with a fever should be checked, unless he or she looks very good, and the fever comes down with Tylenol or Motrin easily. In that case, the baby can be observed and checked later. If the fever is higher than 102.2-102.5° F (39.0-39.1°C), then it is better that the infant gets checked.

## Case #176

Mid-summer

Time: 5:59PM

A three-year-old female toddler

CC: Foreign body ingestion

The toddler has swallowed a penny. She is fine and not complaining. She did not choke on it.

Disposition: Her mother is advised to give her some soft food like white bread and later to observe her stool. If she is having any problems or if she does not pass the penny in the next day or so, then she is to be examined and an x-ray can be obtained. If she prefers, she can be seen sooner for the x-ray. Also, anticipatory guidance is done and preventive measures are mentioned. Avoid leaving coins or tiny objects and medicines accessible to the small children. If the child does not pass the penny later via the stool, the child should be evaluated, and she may also have a blood test for lead.

## Case #177

Mid-summer                                                          Time: 9:21PM

A nine-year-old male child

CC: Fever & right hip pain

The child has been having a fever for four days. His temperature is 103.0°F (39.4°C) today. He is complaining of pain in his right hip. He was seen at the ED four days ago, because he had slipped at the sidewalk and was told he had sprained his ankle on the left side. Since then he has been having a fever and complain of his right hip.

Disposition: The mother is advised to take him to the ED tonight, to be checked. The child with hip pain, and fever should be checked without delay to rule out septic joint or blood/bone infections.

## Case #178

Mid-autumn                                                          Time: 4:50PM

A ten-month-old male infant

CC: Soreness to the tip of penis with bloody spots on diaper

The infant had a cold with slight fever a few days ago, he was seen by a physician and Motrin was advised and the fever subsided. He appears to have soreness to the tip of his penis with a bloody spot on the diaper.

Disposition: The mother is advised to use Bacitracin ointment on the sore tonight, and the infant may be examined tomorrow. The blood could just be due to the prepuce retraction, but because of the previous cold and fever it is prudent to have the child checked.

# Case #179

A three-month-old male infant

CC: Cold & vomiting

The infant has been having a cold and cough for a few days. Normal Saline nose drops were advised. The infant has now been vomiting for the past two or three days. The mother had called today and had spoken to the nurse and was advised to keep giving the infant formula. The infant has normal bowel movements (BMs), has no fever, and is not cranky.

Disposition: The mother is advised to start Pedialyte and to observe. If he cannot retain the Pedialyte, he may be seen at the ED tonight. Rhinovirus infections are the most common cause of cold symptoms and the peak activities of these viruses are in autumn and spring.

# Case #180

A 14-year-old female adolescent

CC: Medicine (Tegretol) refill request

The adolescent has a seizure disorder and needs a refill order for her medicine, Tegretol tablets. She has enough medicine for tonight and tomorrow.

Disposition: Her mother is advised to call her physician tomorrow morning to get the order for the refill because she might need a blood test to obtain the level of the medicine, or the neurologist may want to change the dose of the medicine.

Tegretol (carbamazepine) in 100mg and 200 mg scored tablets or chewable tablets are available options. The indications for its use are generalized tonic–clonic, partial or mixed seizures.

# Case #181

A 16-year-old female adolescent

CC: Abdominal pain & vomiting

The adolescent has been having abdominal pain and vomiting, and no bowel movements for two days. She was seen at the adolescent clinic today and a vaginal exam was done. She received medication via injection and an oral medication. She is sexually active. She continues to complain of abdominal pain and vomiting.

Disposition: She is advised to go to the ED tonight. She has signs of pelvic inflammatory disease (PID), and is not better despite outpatient therapy. Because of the continued pain, she requires more attention and even possible hospitalization to receive intravenous antibiotics. Other causes of pelvic pain in an adolescent female include: ectopic pregnancy, endometriosis, ovarian cysts and masses, ovarian torsion, and dysmenorrhea. That she was seen and received a pelvic exam and then received both an injection (ceftriaxone [Rocephin] for gonorrheal coverage) also an oral medication (azithromycin for chlamydial coverage) implies that she likely had PID.

## Case #182

Date Mid-autumn                                          Time: 9:41PM

A three-month-old male infant

CC: Stuffy nose
The mother states that the baby has had a stuffy nose today and no fever. He is feeding well, voiding well, and he is not cranky.

Disposition: His mother is advised to use Normal Saline nose drops in his nostrils 1-2 drops, three or four times per day and to also use the humidifier in the room, and to observe. If his cold is not getting better in a few days, or if he were to have a fever, he may be examined.

## Case #183

Mid-autumn                                                Time: 11:28PM

An eight-year-old child

CC: Hydrocephalus & shunt, refusing to drink
The child has Hydrocephalus and a VP shunt (ventriculo- peritoneal shunt). He refuses to take his milk and Pediasure.

He vomited once yesterday but there has been no vomiting today. He could retain the Pediasure which was given by syringe. His urine output has been normal.

Disposition: His mother is advised regarding the possibility of a shunt malfunction problem. The mother is instructed to observe, and if he were to vomit again, or is restless, or has any fever, then he should be checked tonight in the ED, otherwise he can be checked tomorrow morning.

## CASE #184

MID-AUTUMN                                                              TIME: 5:37PM

A three-year-old female child

CC: Pink eye, a burning sensation after using eye drops
The child was seen by a physician and received Sulfacetamide 10% ophthalmic drops for pink eye. Her mother has just used one drop in the child's eyes and she complains of a burning sensation.
Disposition: The mother is advised regarding eye hygiene. She is to clean the eyes with sterile water and to observe. If the child cannot tolerate the Sulfacetamide eye drops, then the medicine should be changed.

## CASE #185

LATE AUTUMN                                                             TIME: 8:20PM

A ten-month-old female infant

CC: Fever & diarrhea, on Amoxicillin
The infant had an ear infection 33 days ago. She was seen by a physician and received Bactrim initially, and then the medication was changed to Amoxicillin, because the infant was not getting better. The Amoxicillin was restarted again one week ago, because of fever and continued ear infection. The infant still has a new fever and now has diarrhea.
Disposition: The mother is advised to give her Infants' Tylenol for a temperature ≥100.4°F (38.0°C), offer her clear fluid and Pedialyte, and then to put her on a special diet (rice cereal, apple sauce, plain yogurt, and Lactose-free formula instead of the cow's milk based formula), and to observe. If there is no quick response to Tylenol, then the infant should be examined, because of the possibility of the infection not having responded to Amoxicillin. As the infant has been on 3 courses of oral antibiotics, the infant might need an antibiotic injection (ceftriaxone [Rocephin]). Also, if she were to continue to have recurrent, persistent ear infections, she may need a referral to an ENT (Ear, Nose & Throat) physician, also known as a Head & Neck surgeon.

## CASE #186

TIME: 8:55PM

A nine-week-old male infant

CC: Diarrhea
The infant received his immunizations yesterday. He had DTaP, Comvax (Hemophilus influenzae type B and Hepatitis B), and an IPV (inactivated polio vaccine) immunization. The mother states that the infant has developed diarrhea today and has had two watery and large stools.
Disposition: The mother is advised to give the infant Pedialyte instead of the formula for 4-6 hours and then to observe him and make sure that his condition is improving. The formula can also be changed temporarily to Lactose-free formula if the soft stools persist. Diarrhea is most likely not related to the immunization and is usually virally mediated. The baby can be checked if the stool frequency increases. This call was before the Rotavirus vaccine was available. Now, at nine weeks of age after immunizations there is often a vaccine given which offers protection against Rotavirus, and so diarrhea may indeed be a side effect of the Rotavirus vaccination.

## CASE #187

LATE AUTUMN                                                    TIME: 9:56PM

A four-month-old female infant

CC: Cough & wheezing
The infant has had a history of bronchiolitis in the past. She developed a cough and has been wheezing since yesterday. Albuterol via nebulizer is being used, but she is still having slightly rapid respirations and diarrhea. Mother has been giving the baby only apple juice and white grape juice.
Disposition: The mother is advised to give her Pedialyte instead of juice and to continue the treatments via nebulizer as instructed. In the case that the baby is having difficulty breathing and there are continued rapid respirations, then she should be seen at the ED. It is important not to use fluids like juice and water solely when rehydrating, because there can be a risk of developing hyponatremia (low blood sodium).

## CASE #188

LATE AUTUMN                                                    TIME: 11:17PM

A one-month-old female neonate

CC: Umbilical stump cauterization and now a burn around it

The mother states the baby was seen by her Pediatrician and her umbilical stump was cauterized because of having a wet part. The mother is concerned about the possible burn around it on the surrounding skin.

Disposition: The mother is advised to use Bacitracin ointment on the discolored area three times a day for 3-5 days and to observe. If the skin is just browned, then that will self-resolve. For swelling or redness, the infant can be checked.

## CASE #189

LATE AUTUMN                                                          TIME: 2:08AM

A 23-month-old male toddler

CC: Croupy cough

The child has had a croupy (barky) cough for a few hours. He has had no fever. His father states that the last time that he had the same problem albuterol syrup was prescribed, but the instructions on the bottle have faded.

Disposition: The father is advised to use warm steam in the room, a cool mist humidifier if available, and to give him a ½ teaspoon of albuterol syrup (as sulfate 2mg per 5mL) every 8 hours and to observe. If the child is in distress, he should be seen at the ED.

## CASE #190

LATE AUTUMN                                                          TIME: 9:52AM

A five-month-old female infant

CC: Fever & vomiting

The infant has a temperature of 102.9°F (39.3°C), and has been vomiting. The mother states that the baby was seen by her physician because of the cold symptoms about 5 days ago. The mother is giving her a decongestant medication, but she is not getting better.

Disposition: The mother is advised that the infant should be examined today given new high fevers in the face of an upper respiratory infection. Meanwhile, the mother may give her Infants' Tylenol for fever and offer her clear fluid (Pedialyte and white grape juice), and take her to be checked.

The infant should be examined because she could be developing a secondary bacterial infection. Secondary infections after colds include ear infections and pneumonias, as well as sinus infections.

## CASE #191

A two-year-old male toddler

CC: Coughing & sneezing
The toddler has been coughing and sneezing. He has had no fever, no vomiting, and no mucus from the nose. The child has no history of asthma nor wheezing.
Disposition: The mother is advised to use nose drops (Normal Saline nose drops, one or two drops into the nostrils four times per day for 3-5 days), and the humidifier in the room, and to observe. The mother was Spanish speaking, so advice was given via an interpreter.

## CASE #192

LATE AUTUMN                                                    TIME: 11:05AM

An eleven-month-old male infant

CC: Vomiting after having taken Prednisone & diarrhea
The infant has a history of asthma. She was seen at the ED last week and received a treatment for asthma and Prednisone tablets. The mother states that the infant vomits after taking the Prednisone tablets. He also has been having diarrhea. The mother has been giving him Pedialyte for two days.
Disposition: The mother (Spanish speaking) is advised via an interpreter to use the asthma medicine (albuterol) for his cough, not to give the Prednisone tablets now, and to start Lactose-free formula and observe. If the asthma is worsening or the baby is not voiding at least once every 6 hours, then he may be seen at the ED.

## CASE #193

LATE AUTUMN                                                    TIME: 10:20AM

A two-year-old male toddler

CC: Swollen eyelids & whitish mucus from the eyes
The toddler has minimally swollen eyelids with some whitish mucus from the eyes. He

appears to have some swelling of the face. He has no fever. He urinates well.

Disposition: The mother is advised to clean the eyes, avoid hyper-allergenic foods (egg, chocolate, strawberries, tomato sauce, nuts, and seafood), and observe. If there are signs of infection like fever, worsening redness, swelling, greenish mucus, or eyelash mattering, or if the condition persists then he may be seen in the ED today (weekend call). Otherwise, if he is getting better and not worsening and there is no fever, she may wait until Monday to have him checked at the clinic.

## CASE #194

LATE AUTUMN                                                       TIME: 10:35AM

A four-week-old male neonate

CC: Cough

The mother states that the baby has had a cough for one or two days. He has had no fever, but the mother was giving the baby Infants' Tylenol.

Disposition: The mother is advised not to give the Tylenol and to use Normal Saline nose drops (1-2 drops into the nostrils three to four times per day) and to observe if he continues to cough despite these measures. If the cough persists, he may be examined later today. A neonate with a cough should be checked.

## CASE #195

LATE AUTUMN                                                       TIME: 10:45AM

A 15-year-old male adolescent

CC: Diarrhea while taking Augmentin

The adolescent has an infection of his toe. He was seen two days ago, and received Augmentin 500mg tablet to take three times per day and has been taking the medicine. He has now developed diarrhea.

Disposition: The mother is advised that if the diarrhea is not too frequent or too voluminous, then he should continue the Augmentin 500mg twice per day and she is to put him on a special diet (white rice and starchy foods, applesauce, banana and plain yogurt), and more fluid (Gatorade), and observe. If the diarrhea is severe, then he may need to discontinue the Augmentin and she is to call to possibly change the antibiotic. Diarrhea while on antibiotics is a common side effect as the antibiotics are not specific to the offending organisms and so also destroy the good bacteria of the gastrointestinal tract which can often lead to diarrhea.

# Case #196

A four-month-old male infant

CC: Stuffy nose & touching his ear

The infant has had a stuffy nose and temperature of 100.0ºF. He has been touching his ear. He is feeding well and voiding normally.

Disposition: The mother is advised to use Normal Saline nose drops (one or two drops into the nostrils three or four times per day), and to observe. If the baby were to have a fever (temperature ≥100.4ºF [38.0ºC]) or if worsening ear pains/crankiness, then he may be checked at the ED today (weekend call). Otherwise, if he has no temperature above 100.4ºF (38.0ºC), and is not cranky then they may wait until Monday to have him checked.

# Case #197

Late autumn                                                    Time: 1:51PM

A three-year-old male toddler

CC: Vomiting & diarrhea

The toddler had a fever, diarrhea, and vomiting yesterday. He had two or three episodes of vomiting yesterday. He has had no fever today. He just had a single episode of a small amount of loose stool. However, he is still vomiting.

Disposition: The mother is advised to give him Pedialyte and clear fluid in small amounts and to make sure he can retain it. She may continue this for 4-6 hours and then offer him white rice, applesauce, banana and plain yogurt. The mother is to avoid giving the toddler milk for a few days. If he cannot retain the Pedialyte, he may be seen at the ED. Rotavirus infections are mostly prevalent during the cooler months. Before the introduction of the Rotavirus vaccine, this virus was the most common cause of gastroenteritis in the children.

# Case #198

Late autumn                                                    Time: 2:28PM

A two-year-old female toddler

CC: Fever & sore throat

The child has a fever and a sore throat. She was seen by a physician yesterday and has been told that she has Strep throat, but no antibiotics were given. Children's Motrin was advised for fever and pain. The mother states the child had a high fever at 4:00AM today and that Motrin was given and she has been sleeping more than her usual. She woke up and appears drowsy and refuses to eat because of the sore throat.

Disposition: Given the decreased activity level and the possible Streptococcal pharyngitis diagnosis, the mother is advised to take the child to the ED (weekend call) for reevaluation and throat culture and to receive antibiotic if found to have Strep. A toddler with a positive culture or rapid strep antigen for group A Streptococcal infection and fever should be treated with antibiotics.

## CASE #199

LATE AUTUMN                                                    TIME: 2:40PM

A three-month-old female infant

CC: Constipation

The mother states that the infant has been constipated and has had no bowel movements for 2 or 3 days. She states that the infant is otherwise okay and that she has had no vomiting. She is not cranky and her abdomen is soft.

Disposition: The mother is advised regarding diet; she is to offer the infant small amounts of prune or pear juice (one ounce) diluted in 3-4oz. of water and to also offer her more boiled, cool water to drink, and observe. The mother can also bicycle the legs, massage the abdomen in a clockwise fashion and gently take a rectal temperature using Vaseline to lubricate the thermometer. The mother also is advised that sometimes infants normally have no bowel movement for a few days; if the consistency of the stool is normal, the frequency can be very variable. However, the infant should not be cranky, but should be comfortable and have a soft abdomen and no vomiting. If the infant starts vomiting, or if she were to have any other problem, then the mother is to have the infant examined, but otherwise, she can wait and see how the baby responds to the diluted juice and water and other measures described.

## CASE #200

LATE AUTUMN                                                    TIME: 3:41PM

A two-year-old female toddler

CC: Cough & asthma, on prednisone with a question about medicine

The child has a history of bronchial asthma and is on albuterol inhalation solution via nebulizer and prednisone 20mg tablets, one and a half tablets on first day then to be increased to one and a half tablets twice per day, then 3 tablets once per day. The child has no fever, and no vomiting, but still has a cough. The child is on Amoxicillin for the ear infection.

Disposition: The mother is advised and the prednisone dose is adjusted according to the child's weight which is 38 lbs. It is to be given 2mg/kg daily for 3 to 5 days and she is to be observed.

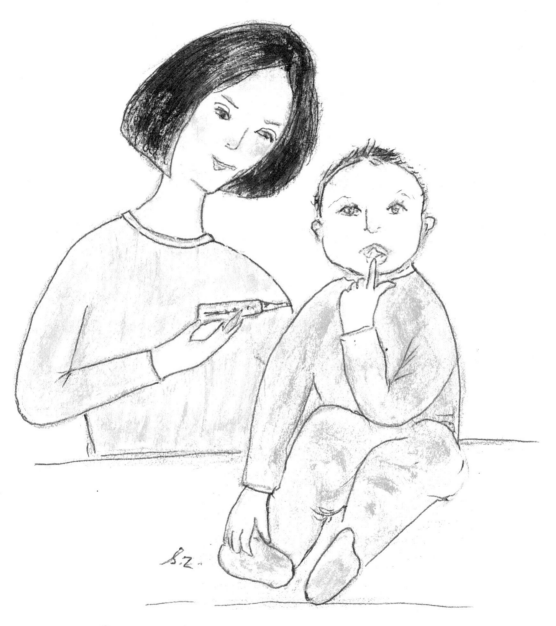

Case #175

A 10-month-old infant with fever

# Chapter Five

---

## Case #201

Late autumn                                                          Time: 5:09PM

A two-year-old female toddler

CC: Asthma & medication question

The child is an asthmatic. She is in no distress, but her mother inquires if she can give her a cough syrup besides the asthma medicine.

Disposition: Mother is advised that she may give her plain Robitussin cough syrup, ½ teaspoon three times per day, for 3-5 days. While that was my advice and standard of care then, nowadays cough and cold medicine are not advisable for children 6 years and under. The mother is advised to use the asthma medicine (albuterol) via the spacer to open the airways and alleviate her cough. She is to continue to use the albuterol every four to six hours until the cough subsides. The mother is also advised to give extra fluid as this helps to moisturize the mucous membranes, liquefy secretions, and works as an expectorant.

## Case #202

Late autumn                                                          Time: 5:22PM

A nine-month-old female infant

CC: Fever & loose bowel movements

The infant has a fever. Her temperature was taken about 10 minutes ago and was 103.0ºF (39.4ºC) and Infants' Tylenol has been given to her. She has no cold symptoms and no vomiting. Her bowel movements are loose, and she has had three such stools today. Her appetite has not been good for the past 2-3 days. She probably had a slight fever yesterday.

Disposition: The mother is advised to give her more fluids (water, juice, soup) and if she is responding to Tylenol and she does not look sick, then she is to be observed at home and may be checked tomorrow in clinic. Given that there is a source for the fever (diarrhea, which is most commonly due to a virus), as long as the fever can be controlled, and the oral intake is adequate, the infant can be seen the following day. Otherwise, if the fever is not responding to antipyretic, or if the infant is ill-appearing or with pain (fussiness), or if there is any blood in stool, then she is to be seen at the ED tonight.

## Case #203

Late autumn                                                    Time: 7:33PM

A 14-month old female infant

CC: Vomiting

The infant vomited once last night after taking her milk. She vomited twice this afternoon. There is neither blood nor bile in the emesis. She is teething with several teeth coming in and has had two loose bowel movements today. She has no fever but, likely because of teething, her temperature has been 100.3-100.4°F (37.9-38.0°C) for the past few days.

Disposition: The mother is advised to give her Pedialyte and clear fluid (white grape juice, flat ginger ale) for 6-12 hours and dietary advice (rice cereal, applesauce, and banana) is also given. The child is to be observed and if she were to continue to vomit, if her urinary pattern changes, or if there is fever greater than 102.2°F (39.0°C), then she may be checked at that point.

## Case #204

Late autumn                                                    Time: 7:45PM

A 23-month-old female toddler

CC: Fever & medication question

The child has a slight fever, her temperature is 100.4-100.7°F (38.0-38.1°C). She also has a slight cough. Her mother would like to know how much Tylenol she can give her.

Disposition: The mother is advised to give her Tylenol for a temperature ≥100.4°F (38.0°C), and that the dose of Tylenol (Children's Tylenol syrup, 160mg per 5 mL)

for her is about 4 mL every four to six hours for fever. The child weighs 23 pounds, or about 10.5 kg. The dose of the acetaminophen (Tylenol) is 10 to 15mg per kg of body weight per dose, with a maximum of 75mg/kg/day.

## CASE #205

A three-year-old male toddler

CC: Fever
The toddler has a fever and a slight runny nose. His temperature is 104.0°F (40.0°C). He vomited twice today. The vomiting was after his having taken the Tylenol. His last bowel movements were 2 days ago, and was greenish.
Disposition: The mother is advised to give him Children's Motrin (100mg/5mL, one and a half teaspoons every six to eight hours) or Children's Tylenol (acetaminophen, 120mg rectal suppository) for the fever, to give him clear fluid (Pedialyte, white grape juice, flat ginger ale), and to observe.
If he continues with high fevers and vomiting, and cannot keep the fluid down, then he is to be seen at the ED. The dose of the ibuprofen (Motrin) is 5 to 10mg/kg/dose, every 6 to 8 hours, with a maximum of 40mg/kg/day.

## CASE #206

A 14-month-old female infant

CC: Runny nose & diarrhea
The infant has been having a runny nose for about 2-3 weeks. She has been having diarrhea for 3 days. She has had no fever. She tugs on her ear sometimes, but she also has earrings.
Disposition: The mother is advised to give the infant Pedialyte and clear fluid (white grape juice, flat ginger ale), and dietary advice (rice cereal or soft well-cooked rice, applesauce, banana, plain yogurt) is given. If the condition persists, or if she has a fever ≥102.2°F (39.0°C), then the infant is to be examined.

## CASE #207

A 27-day-old male neonate

CC: Maternal fever & breast problem
The baby is taking breastmilk and is fine, but the mother has soreness of her nipples and pain and a possible fever.
Disposition: The mother is advised to be checked by her own physician and to meanwhile extract her milk with the breast pump. The baby is taking formula too.


## CASE #208

A ten-month-old female infant

CC: Fever & nose bleeding
The infant has a history of recurrent ear infection. The last episode of her ear infection was 2 days ago, she was seen and received Zithromax, which she just started yesterday. The infant has high fever today. Her temperature is 103.0°F (39.4°C). She has nose bleeding as well. She has no vomiting. She has been very cranky.
Disposition: The mother is advised to take the baby to the ED to be reexamined, given the delay in treating the infant, symptoms that are worsening instead of improving while on antibiotics, current high fever and crankiness and the child's personal history. It is better for this child to be checked and perhaps to receive either antibiotic by injection or another type of antibiotic, since it appears she is not responding to Zithromax.
The physician might opt to give the antibiotic more time to work, but given the delay in care, high fever, and fussiness, the child may be rechecked.


## CASE #209

A 16-year-old male adolescent

CC: Eye injury & fever
The adolescent had an eye injury 4 days ago, he was hospitalized for 2 days. He was discharged with an eye patch and prednisolone eye drops. His mother has a question regarding his two follow-up appointments that he has tomorrow morning. She also states he has temperature of 100.2°F (37.8°C) and is complaining about his throat. His sibling presently has a stomach virus.
Disposition: The mother is advised to give him Tylenol (one adult Tylenol 325mg

tablet, every 4 to 6 hour for fever or pain) and to offer him more fluid (water, juice, soup), and to observe. She may just keep the appointments tomorrow morning as a temperature less than 100.4°F (38.0°C) is not considered to be a true fever. With the sibling as an ill contact and sore throat, a low-grade temperature is most likely unrelated to the eye condition, but possibly related to a forthcoming viral infection.

## Case #210

A ten-month-old male infant

CC: Dietary question
The infant has a history of bronchiolitis and is currently under treatment. The mother has a question regarding whether eggs induce asthma. She would like to start giving the baby eggs.
There is no history of egg allergy in the past or in the family.
Disposition: Egg white is a hyper-allergenic food and if has not already been tried, it should not be introduced until after the child's first birthday. Likewise, it is better to hold-off on introducing new foods when a child is acutely ill with a respiratory infection, as it will be difficult to ascertain if the child is having a reaction to the new food or if the intercurrent illness is responsible for any reactions. Since the time when I gave my advice, the recommendations for introduction of egg into the infant's diet have changed and so it would have been permissible to introduce egg, first yolk and then the white, into an infant's diet for whom allergy is not suspected. Again, as this particular child is ill, it would be better to wait until the child is not ill.

## Case #211

A 17-month-old male toddler

CC: Fever
The toddler has been having a fever, temperature of 103.0-104.0°F (39.4-40.0°C) for the last 3-4 days. Tylenol has been given, but the fever quickly returns. He has been cranky and has lost his appetite. On one occasion, he has vomited the Tylenol. He also had one loose bowel movement with odor. He also has a history of vomiting and diarrhea 2 weeks ago, and was seen at the ED then.
Disposition: Given the irritability, more than 3 days of high fever, and prolonged

symptoms, the mother is advised to have the child checked. She should also push fluid like Pedialyte, white grape juice, flat ginger ale and give him Children's Motrin (100mg/5mL) every 6 to 8 hours or Children's Tylenol (160mg/5mL) every 4 hours as needed for the fever.

## CASE #212

LATE AUTUMN                                                    TIME: 1:43PM

A seven-week-old male infant

CC: Feeding difficulty
The mother states that the baby is taking the formula less than he was before. He is on breastmilk and Enfamil with Iron. He has no fever, no vomiting, and no diarrhea. The urine output and bowel patterns have been normal. He is breastfeeding well.
Disposition: The mother is advised that the infant is most likely taking more breastmilk and so might need less formula for that reason and to also look inside the baby's mouth for any lesions. Frequent feeding is advised, and the baby is to be observed. If the mother suspects that the baby continues to have a problem, then the baby can be checked tomorrow. If there is a change in the urine output, a fever (a rectal temperature ≥100.4ºF [38.0ºC]), or if the breastfeeding is also not going well, then the baby may be checked sooner.

## CASE #213

LATE AUTUMN                                                    TIME: 3: 47PM

A ten-month-old female infant

CC: Rash
The mother states that the baby had a history of oral thrush about 9-10 days ago, and likewise he had an ear infection 4 days ago. She was seen and is on Amoxicillin. The infant has now developed a rash all over her body and she thinks that it may be related to a new apple juice that she just started for her last night. The baby is constipated and had no bowel movements for a few days but she has no vomiting and is not cranky.
Disposition: The mother is advised to use Calamine lotion on the rash, and was advised to give the baby water to drink. She may also offer juices like prune and pear juice and she is to offer her oatmeal instead of rice cereal for the constipation. If she truly suspects that the rash is related to the specific apple juice, it is best not to give her that kind of apple juice. When any new food or juice is introduced into her diet, just

offer her a small amount in the beginning and make sure she is not allergic to it and does not show any reaction. Do not start anything new when she has a rash, or she is sick, and take her to be checked tomorrow. A rash related to an underlying virus is also a possibility. A reaction to Amoxicillin may also be considered, and the Amoxicillin can be stopped until she is evaluated tomorrow.

## Case #214

Late autumn                                                       Time: 5:16PM

A two-year-old male toddler

CC: Poor appetite & refusing to drink
The mother states that the child had an ear infection 3 days ago. He was seen by physician and is on Amoxicillin and Tylenol for fever. The child appears to be getting better. He has no fever but his appetite is not good and he does not want to drink. He urinated a while ago.
Disposition: The mother is advised to let him drink (water, juice, and flat ginger ale) sip by sip and to observe him. If he urinates every 6-8 hours he is likely not so dehydrated. If he keeps having the problem, he may be checked tomorrow.

## Case #215

Late autumn                                                       Time: 5:41PM

A three-year-old male toddler

CC: Fever
The mother states that the child has had a fever since last night. His temperature was 102.0°F (38.8°C) last night and Tylenol was given. He has had no vomiting and no cold symptoms. His appetite is not good, but he drinks well and urinates well. His temperature is 103.3°F (39.6°C) this afternoon.
Disposition: The mother is advised to give him Children's Tylenol (160mg/5mL, one teaspoon every 4 hours) or Children's Motrin (100mg/5mL, 6mL every 6 to 8 hours) for fever, and to push fluid (water, juice, flat ginger ale, soup). If he looks sick and continues to have a high fever, he may be seen tonight, otherwise he may be seen tomorrow morning.
Human herpes virus 6 (Roseola) infection causes high fever, and happens mostly in toddlers, and may occur throughout the year. The young child with a high fever should be checked.

## Case #216

A one-month-old male neonate

CC: Whitish spots in the mouth (thrush)
His mother just noticed that the baby has a few whitish spots in the mouth.
Disposition: The mother is advised to call in the morning and take the baby to be seen tomorrow to receive medication for the treatment of oral thrush.

## Case #217

A three-month-old female infant

CC: Eye redness & swelling
According to the father, the baby's right eye appears red and slightly swollen and this started today in the afternoon. She has had no fever, no vomiting. No diarrhea and no other problem. She is well-appearing, feeding well and with normal urine output.
Disposition: Her father is advised to clean the eyes with sterile water tonight and to call and take the baby to be examined tomorrow. Given the young age of the baby, a thorough examination is warranted even if conjunctivitis (pink eye) is suspected.

## Case #218

An eight-month-old female infant

CC: Cold symptoms
The infant has had a cold for about seven days. She has been having a slight fever off-and-on since about 5 days ago; now, she has a slight cough and phlegm and her temperature is 100.0°F (37.7°C). Her mother has been giving her Pediacare and Infants' Tylenol.
Disposition: The mother is advised to use Normal Saline nose drops in her nostrils (1-2 drops, 3-4 times per day), and to offer the baby more fluid (water, juice, broth). She is to call and take the baby in to be examined tomorrow, if the cold is not getting better given the symptom duration.

# Case #219

Time: 12:31AM

A five-year-old male child

CC: Asthma & pneumonia

The child is a known asthmatic who has been seen at the ED twice in the past 2 days, and has received asthma treatment via nebulizer as well as prednisone at the hospital. The mother has been told that he has pneumonia, and the child is on erythromycin at home. He is not on any other liquid medicine for his cough. He has been coughing a great deal and sometimes has difficulty breathing. He is now asleep and breathing well. The mother is asking for cough syrup.

Disposition: The mother is advised that she should use the child's albuterol MDI via spacer, 2 puffs every four hours and that this should ameliorate the cough. She should also continue the erythromycin as instructed. He does not need any separate cough syrup. The mother also is advised to offer him extra fluid to drink to help liquefy the secretions.

# Case #220

Early winter                                                      Time: 4:59AM

A three-year-old male toddler

CC: Headache & right eye pain

The child woke up this morning and has been complaining of a headache. He complains of pain at the top of his head and at the right side of his head and that his right eye hurts. He has no fever and no vomiting. He has been having cold and mucus from his nose for the past few days. His mother has given him 2 Children's Tylenol chewable tablets (80mg Tylenol chewable tablets) this morning.

Disposition: The mother is advised that the child should be checked today. The child might just have a viral infection, but given worsening symptoms, he can be seen to make sure is not developing a secondary bacterial infection. The child who has been having a cold with thick mucus, and then develops headache and eye pain, should be examined.

# Case #221

Early winter                                                      Time: 5:41PM

A six-week-old male neonate

CC: Cold symptoms

The baby has had a cold and cough for 2 days. His temperature was not taken, but he appears to be warm. He has no vomiting. He is feeding well, and voiding a normal amount.

Disposition: His mother is advised to take a rectal temperature and that if the infant has any fever (rectal temperature ≥100.4°F [38.0°C]) or if he is coughing often, then he should be seen tonight, otherwise she is to use Normal Saline nose drops (one or two drops into his nostrils three or four times per day), and a humidifier and to call tomorrow morning to have the baby checked.


## CASE #222

EARLY WINTER                                                     TIME: 7: 35PM

A 20-month-old male toddler

CC: Vomiting & weakness

The toddler had a prolonged cold and an ear infection about 10 days ago. He was seen 10 days ago, and received Amoxicillin. The mother states she lost the bottle of Amoxicillin, and received another bottle of medicine. The child was doing well but has developed vomiting this afternoon and appears to be weak.

Disposition: The mother is advised to start Pedialyte immediately and that if he is still weak despite her pushing fluid, then he is to be seen at the ED.


## CASE #223

EARLY WINTER                                                     TIME: 8:05PM

A 26-month-old male toddler

CC: Fever & diarrhea

His father states that the child has been having a fever off-and-on for 2 days. He has had loose bowel movements three times today. He has not had any vomiting. His father gave him Children's Motrin about 5 hours ago, and he has no fever now.

Disposition: The father is advised to give him Pedialyte and clear fluid that is non-sugary. He is not to give too much fruit juice as the hyperosmolar sugars (fructose and sorbitol) from juices may make diarrhea worse. He is to observe him and if he continues to have a fever, especially if higher than 102.2°F (39.0°C), then he is to have him examined tomorrow.

## Case #224

A four-year-old male child

CC: Vomiting & diarrhea

The child has a fever, diarrhea, and vomiting all starting today. He vomited three times today, and has had three watery stools today. His temperature was 103.0°F (39.4°C) and he received Children's Tylenol.

Disposition; His mother is advised to give him Pedialyte and clear fluid. If he cannot retain the Pedialyte, has blood in the stool, or has severe abdominal pain, then he is to be seen at the ED. Rotavirus infection is more common in the cooler seasons and in children attending daycare.

## Case #225

Early winter                                          Time: 8:23PM

A six-year-old male child

CC: Fever & ear pain

The child has been having a fever off-and-on and has been complaining of ear pain since about 2 days ago. He had a temperature of 102.0°F (38.8°C) two days ago, Children's Motrin was given and he was feeling better. He has had no vomiting and he has not yet been checked.

Disposition: The mother is advised that the child should be checked. If he feels better with Tylenol or Motrin and his pain is controlled, she may wait until tomorrow and have him checked then. The child with fever and earache most probably has an ear infection. He should be checked and then receive proper antibiotics.

## Case #226

Early winter                                          Time: 8:34PM

An 18-month-old female toddler

CC: Eye concern

The child was seen at an eye clinic today and eye drops were used to dilate her pupils. Her mother states that the child's pupils are still widely opened. The child is doing well otherwise.

Disposition: The mother is reassured. The effect of the cycloplegics used at the eye doctor, can cause prolonged dilation of the pupil. When the pupils are dilated, exposure to strong light should be avoided.

## Case #227

A 20-month-old male toddler

CC: Diarrhea & vomiting
The child had diarrhea and vomiting since about 4 days ago. His mother gave him clear fluid and the vomiting has stopped 2 days ago, but he still has diarrhea. He has had several loose bowel movements (BMs). His mother has been giving him milk today.
Disposition: The mother is advised to stop the milk, and to give him Pedialyte and foods like white rice, applesauce, banana and other fluid besides Pedialyte, like water and flat ginger ale. When his diarrhea is getting better and he wants milk, please offer him Lactaid milk for a few days. If there is blood in the stool, a marked decrease in urine output, or severe episodic abdominal pains, then the child should be checked. Otherwise, she can expect the viral illness to last up to 8 days or so.

## Case #228

A one-year-old female infant

CC: Rash
Her father states that the child has developed a rash on her trunk and back since yesterday. She was on Amoxicillin because of an ear infection recently but not currently. She had a high fever for 3 or 4 days, and developed the rash when she had no fever. She is otherwise well.
Disposition: The father is advised to use Calamine lotion on the rash and to have the infant examined tomorrow.
The possibility of having Roseola Infantum or an allergic rash is explained, and is to be determined after the examination.
The responsible virus for Roseola infection is human herpes virus 6 (HHV-6). The main clinical manifestation is high fever for about 4-5 days and erythematous maculopapular rash appears after the fever resolves. Roseola infection predominantly develops between the ages of 6 months to 3 years. The infections occur throughout the

year without a seasonal pattern.

## Case #229

A six-month-old male infant

CC: Fever & cold symptoms
The infant has had a cold and fever. He has had no vomiting. He has been congested. He is feeding well and has a normal urine output.
Disposition: The mother is advised to take the temperature, and give him Infants' Tylenol every four to six hours for temperatures ≥100.4°F (38.0°C), to use Normal Saline nose drops in his nostrils (one or two drops into the nostrils, three or four times per day) and to offer him fluid (juice, water and his formula). If he has a fever ≥102.2°F (39.0°C), then he may be examined tomorrow.

## Case #230

A three-year-old female child

CC: Earache
The child had a fever, cold and vomiting 4 days ago, she was seen at the ED and Children's Tylenol was advised and she has been fine. Tonight, she has complained about her ear.
Disposition: The father is advised to call and take the child to be examined, at the pediatric clinic tomorrow morning.
A dose of Children's Motrin (100mg/5mL) is also advised, as Motrin lasts up to 8 hours and acts as an anti-inflammatory as well as a pain medicine, and so may better help the inflammation in the ear.

## Case #231

A one-year-old male infant

CC: Fever & cough
The infant has had a cold and cough and vomiting on occasion after coughing. He

has developed a fever tonight. His temperature is 102.6°F (39.2°C) and his mother just gave him Infants' Tylenol. His sibling currently has Strep throat. The child is an asthmatic.

Disposition: His mother is advised to give him fluid (juice, broth, flat ginger ale) and his asthma medicine (albuterol) via nebulizer. Since she just gave him Tylenol, she may observe to see if he is getting better and that the fever is coming down. If so, then he is to be checked in the morning at the clinic. For any respiratory concerns, or if he is not responding to the albuterol, then he may be seen sooner at the ED.

## CASE #232

EARLY WINTER                                                        TIME: 6:51AM

A six-month-old male infant

CC: Fever & cough

The infant has a fever and cough. He was examined five days ago, and Motrin was advised. His temperature is 103.6°F (39.7°C) now and his mother just gave him Infants' Tylenol.

Disposition: The mother is advised to offer him more fluids (water, juice), to undress him to help bring the temperature down, and to bring him in to be checked early this morning. The most commonly responsible viruses for upper respiratory infections of infants include rhinovirus, influenza and parainfluenza viruses and respiratory syncytial virus (RSV).

## CASE #233

EARLY SPRING                                                        TIME: 7:01PM

An eight-month-old male infant

CC: Fever & vomiting

The infant has had one day of fever and vomiting. He is exclusively breastfed. His temperature is 101.0°F (38.3°C) and his mother has given him Infants' Tylenol, and he appears to be getting better. His vomiting is also better. He has had no bowel movements for 2 days.

Disposition: The mother is advised to give him Pedialyte and observe him. Well-appearing infants with low grade temperatures likely due to viral etiologies, can be observed. If he were to have a high fever ≥102.2-102.5°F (39.0-39.1°C), or a decrease in urinary output, then he may be checked sooner. However, if he is improving, he may be checked on Monday (weekend call).

## Case #234

A two-week-old female neonate

CC: Medication error
The newborn's mother is HIV positive and the baby is on AZT. The mother accidentally gave the baby an extra dose of the medication (the next dose was given too soon by mistake). The infant is doing well.
Disposition: The mother is advised to observe and skip the next dose. Zidovudine (AZT) was given to the newborn infants with maternal Human immunodeficiency virus infection to decrease the rate of maternal to infant transmission of HIV. The dose of Zidovudine for the full-term neonate is 2mg/kg, 4 times per day for the first 6 weeks of life. Alternatively, we could have also contacted poison control 1-800-222-1222 to see if they had any further instructions.

## Case #235
Early spring                                                        Time: 12:37AM

A seven-week-old male infant

CC: A lump at the immunization site
The infant has had swelling at the site of his HiB immunization which was given 2 days ago, he has had no fever and no redness on that area. He is in no pain and is otherwise well.
Disposition: The mother is advised to use a cold compress on the swelling for 10-15 minutes a few times per day and to observe. She is to call us for signs of infection (pain, redness, fever).

## Case #236
Early spring                                                        Time: 7:23AM

A 2-year-old female toddler

CC: Fever
The child has been having a fever for the past 3 days. Motrin and Tylenol have been

given but the toddler continues to have a high fever. Her temperature is 103.3ºF (39.6ºC) this morning. She has no vomiting, she is not drinking well, and has not had a bowel movement today.

Disposition: The mother is advised to take the child to be examined today. A child with a high fever not responding to antipyretics should be checked. Meanwhile, offer her fluid (water, juices like pear juice, apricot juice and flat ginger ale) and continue Children's Tylenol 160mg/5mL (one teaspoon every four hours for temperature of ≥100.4ºF [38.0ºC]) or Children's Motrin 100mg/5mL (6mL every six to eight hours for temperature of ≥102.2ºF [39.0ºC]).

## Case #237

Early spring                                          Time: 11:00AM

A 17-year-old female adolescent

CC: Asthma

The adolescent is having an exacerbation of her asthma. Her asthma medication was used via nebulizer but she is not improving. She has no Prednisone at home.

Disposition: The adolescent is advised to repeat her albuterol via nebulizer in 20 minutes, and if not improving, then she is to be examined at the ED.

## Case #238

Early spring                                          Time: 11:06AM

A six-year-old male child

CC: Fever & dental caries (cavities)

The child has history of cleft lip and cleft palate. He has a large dental cavity in a molar tooth and complains of pain there, and has a fever since last night. Children's Motrin was given earlier, but it has not helped.

Disposition: The mother is advised to repeat the Motrin if six hours has passed since the prior dose, and if it is working she may wait until tomorrow to have the child seen. Otherwise, he may need to be seen today if the fever and pain cannot be controlled.

She should give him Children's Motrin 100mg/5mL, two teaspoons every six to eight hours.

## Case #239

A three-year-old female child

CC: Earache
The child has had an earache since last night. Her mother gave her Children's Motrin which helped temporarily. However, she has now developed pain again, and a slight fever.
Disposition: The mother is advised to try Motrin 100mg/5mL, 6mL, every six to eight hours and to observe to see if the child is better. If so, she may be seen tomorrow morning. The child has signs of an ear infection and may need an antibiotic. The first-choice antibiotic for the child below 5 years of age is Amoxicillin 80-90mg/kg per day divided into 2-3 doses (for Acute Otitis Media). Some viral infections produce clear secretions behind the tympanic membrane which also cause an earache. It is advisable to have the ears checked in order not to receive unnecessary antibiotics.

## Case #240

Early spring                                                          Time: 7:48PM

A two-year-old female child

CC: Streptococcal pharyngitis & vomiting
The child has been vomiting. She was seen at the hospital 3 days ago, and Pedialyte was advised. Today she received a call that her throat culture was positive for Streptococcal pharyngitis.
Disposition: The mother is taking the child to the hospital to be treated and she is asking for physician approval. She is calling and seeking an injectable form of treatment since the child is vomiting and unable to keep anything down.
Positive throat culture for group A streptococcal (GAS) pharyngitis or strep throat in a symptomatic child should be treated with an oral or injectable penicillin, or if better tolerated, oral Amoxicillin for 10 days.

## Case #241

Early spring                                                          Time: 8:37PM

A three-year-old male child

CC: Daytime wetting (diurnal enuresis)

His mother states the child has been wetting his pants for the past three days, which is new for him. He has had no fever.

Disposition: The mother is advised to take the child to the clinic in the morning for a urine test. With a simple urine test we can rule out urinary tract infection, diabetes mellitus, diabetes insipidus and other pathologic conditions; and we may also do other tests if required.

If the urine test and physical examination are negative, the condition (enuresis) or polyuria could be related to emotional stress. We should inquire if the child has been drinking a lot of fluid or if anything unusual has happened in the past few days in the family's life.

## CASE #242

EARLY SPRING                                                TIME: 8:38PM

A four-month-old male infant

CC: Constipation (hard stools)

The infant has had constipation since last night; he has no vomiting and no other problem.

Disposition: The mother is advised to offer the baby water to drink and to offer him diluted prune juice (one ounce of juice in 4oz. of water) and to observe.

Juices like prune, apricot, pear, and peach (containing the hyperosmolar sugars fructose and sorbitol) help infants to have bowel movements. However, one should be cautious when giving these to small infants, as they may lead to the development of diarrhea.

## CASE #243

EARLY SPRING                                                TIME: 4:50PM

A seven-year-old male child

CC: Vomiting in a child with cerebral palsy (CP)

The child has cerebral palsy and is a special needs child. He takes nutrients via NG (nasogastric) tube. He vomited twice today, once occurring while he was at school.

Disposition: The mother is advised to take his temperature and observe his bowel movement. Pedialyte and clear fluid are to be given via NG tube for one or two feedings and the child is to be observed. The child is to be checked in the morning if required.

## Case #244

A two-year-old male toddler

CC: Diarrhea

The child had diarrhea 2 days ago, and his diarrhea was improving. However, he developed more diarrhea again after having had milk, and eating an apple, orange and a hotdog today.

Disposition: The mother is advised regarding the diet and asked not to start the cow's milk soon after diarrhea. She may instead offer Lactaid milk in a couple days. She is to give him soft and well-cooked rice and other starchy foods as well as applesauce, banana, and plain yogurt. Also, she is to avoid giving him raw fruits and vegetables for a few days after the diarrhea to expedite his recovery.

## Case #245

An eight-month-old male infant

CC: Fever

The infant is a special needs child who has had a history of congenital herpes (HSV) encephalitis/meningitis. He was seen at the ED two days ago, and received Valium 5mg and has been sleepy since. He was also seen by the physician for children with special needs yesterday, and his mother was given advice. Today, he has had a slight fever and has been at his baseline level of fussiness and is less sleepy.

Disposition: His mother is advised to give him Infants' Tylenol or Children's Motrin (100mg/5mL) for the fever and if he is increasingly cranky, and is on Valium for this reason, he may be given a half dose of the Valium and be observed. For high fevers or increasing fussiness not better with the Valium, he should be rechecked. Otherwise, in the morning, the mother should please place a call into the Special Needs Clinic physician's office to set up a follow-up exam.

## Case #246

A nine-month-old female infant

CC: Fever & diarrhea

The infant has been having diarrhea and fever for three days. Her mother had called her pediatrician and was advised to give her Pedialyte and clear fluid and she was getting better, but her mother was worried and took her to be examined at the hospital today anyway. She just had called again to be reassured.

Disposition: She is advised that after the clear fluid she may start Lactose-free formula and cereal and other starches as well.

CASE #247
EARLY SPRING                                                  TIME: 6:29PM

A three-month-old female infant

CC: Scalp rash (cradle cap)

The infant has cradle cap and seborrhea of scalp. She also has dry patches on her skin and to back of her neck. Her mother has a history of eczema.

Disposition: The mother is advised regarding the diet (not to start solid foods too early). She is also advised regarding the type of formula (instead of a cow's milk based formula, she could try a soy based formula, and if the skin condition is not getting any better she may even try a protein hydrolysate formula like Nutramigen). Advice is also given regarding skin care (she is to use a mild soap like Dove Sensitive Skin to bathe the baby, not to bathe her too often, and to avoid using soap on her face). Also, the mother was advised to use baby oil on the scalp through the night and wash the scalp with baby shampoo in the morning. She can also use Selsun Blue shampoo once a week.

CASE #248
EARLY SPRING                                                  TIME: 1:21AM

A 17-month-old female toddler

CC: Cold symptoms & gagging

The child has been having a cold for about four days. She also has been having yellowish phlegm. She woke up gagging and trying to vomit the phlegm. It appears that her forehead is warm and that her hands are cold and shaking.

Disposition: The mother is advised to take her temperature and give her Children's Tylenol every four to six hours or Children's Motrin 100mg/5mL every six to eight hours for fever. She should also offer her more clear fluid (water, juice, soup and flat ginger ale) to drink. She is to have her examined today, given the gagging event.

A 17-month-old male toddler

CC: Fever & diarrhea
The child has been having diarrhea for four days. He had fever of 102.0ºF (38.8ºC) yesterday afternoon. Children's Tylenol was given at that time and he now has temperature of 103.0ºF (39.4ºC). He also has mucus in the stool. There is no blood in the stool.
Disposition: The mother is advised to give him Children's Motrin (100mg/5mL) for fever, and clear fluid and Pedialyte, and have him checked later today, in clinic.
Rotavirus infection associated with fever and diarrhea is prevalent in cooler months and mostly in infants and toddlers and can cause dehydration.
Shigella species can also induce foodborne bacterial diarrhea associated with high fever sand mucoid stools. With Shigella, there may or may not be blood in the stool. This agent should also be kept in mind.

A five-month-old female infant

CC: Eyelid swelling
The infant has slight swelling below her right eye today. She has no other problem, no fever, no eye discharge nor redness. The mother denies any new food having been introduced to the infant's diet, nor did she notice any insect exposure.
Disposition: The mother is advised to use a cold compress on the swelling for 10-15 minutes a few times per day and observe to see that it is improving. The child may be checked, however if the condition persists.

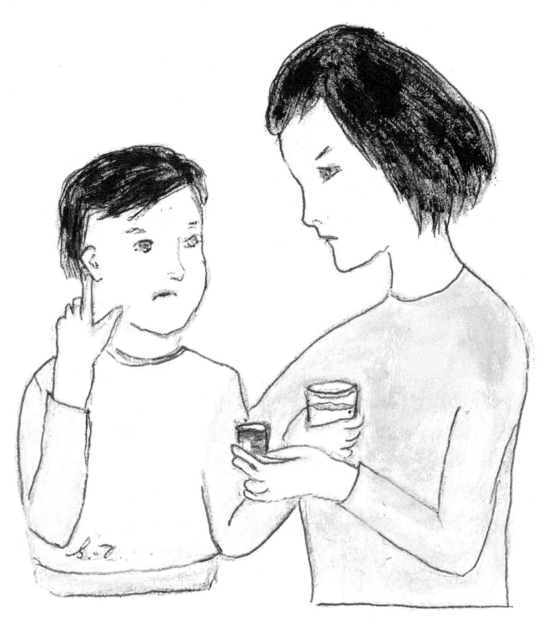

Case #225

A 6-year-old child with fever and complains of his ear

# Chapter Six

～∾～

## Case #251

Time: 1:10AM

A 24-day-old male neonate

CC: Diarrhea

The neonate has had diarrhea for one or two days. He has no fever and no vomiting. He has been on Enfamil with iron formula. He had several bowel movements which were initially voluminous but is now having small amounts of softer stools.

Disposition: The mother is advised via interpreter to give the baby Pedialyte for 6 to 12 hours. She may then start a Lactose-free formula for a 2-week period. If he keeps having copious diarrhea, develops any fever (rectal temperature ≥100.4°F (38.0°C), has any blood in stool, is fussy/in pain or is not voiding every 6-8 hours or so, then he should be examined at the hospital (ED). If not, then they can follow up with their pediatrician should the watery stools persists.

## Case #252

Mid-spring Time: 1:40PM

A two-year-old male toddler

CC: Fever

The child has been having a fever off-and-on for 2-3 days. His temperature was not taken prior to today. No medicine has been given for the fever. Currently his temperature is 103.1°F (39.5°C) and he has been having a runny nose. He has had no vomiting.

Disposition: The mother is advised to give him ibuprofen (Children's Motrin 100mg/5mL, one teaspoon every six to eight hours) for fever, offer him more fluid (juice, soup, flat ginger ale) to drink and to observe him. If he keeps having a high fever, then he is to be examined today.

## Case #253

Mid-spring                                                    Time: 3:57PM

A four-month-old female infant

CC: Fever

The infant has a fever; her temperature is 103.0°F (39.4°C). The fever started today. Her grandmother suspects that the infant has an ear infection "because the wax is coming out of her ears." She has no vomiting.

Disposition: The grandmother is advised to give her infants' acetaminophen (Infants' Tylenol) 40mg, every four to six hours for temp ≥100.4°F (38.0°C), to offer her fluid (water, diluted apple juice, formula), and to have her examined today. Given the young age of the infant (four months old) and the high temperature (≥102.2°F [39.0°C]), it is important to have the child checked soon.

## Case #254

Spring                                                        Time: 7:30PM

A seven-year-old male child

CC: Asthma medicine refill request

The child has a history of asthma and needs refills of his asthma medicine. His mother left us the phone number of her pharmacy and is asking us to call in the medicine. I called and according to the pharmacist, the mother did not wait for the refill and decided to take the child to the doctor to be seen tonight and so no longer needs refills now.

These types of calls occur sometimes during the night call, so the on-call physician should be aware of them.

## Case #255

Spring                                                        Time: 10:15PM

A 14-month-old male infant

CC: Diarrhea & vomiting
The child has developed diarrhea and non-bloody and non-bilious vomiting that started this evening. He has no fever. There is neither blood nor mucus in stool.
Disposition: I recommended that the mother start Pedialyte in small amounts (1-2 oz.) to be given in short intervals, (every 20 minutes), and to make sure he can retain that. Thereafter, she may continue the Pedialyte for 6 to 12 hours. If the infant cannot keep the Pedialyte down, then the mother may have him checked tonight. Otherwise, he may be examined tomorrow.
A fourteen-month-old infant who cannot retain oral rehydration fluid should be checked soon.

## CASE #256
SPRING                                                           TIME: 10:29PM

A two-year-old male toddler

CC: Fever & pain in the chest and stomach
The child has a subjective fever which started this evening and complains that "it hurts" while pointing to his chest and stomach.
The mother states that she cannot take his temperature and she suspects the child might have accidentally ingested something.
Disposition: The mother is advised if she truly suspects possible foreign body ingestion, then she should take him to be checked tonight.
Accidental ingestion can be dangerous especially if medications, batteries or magnets are ingested. Coins can also be problematic if they get stuck in the upper esophagus or airway.

## CASE #257
SPRING                                                           TIME: 12:13AM

A six-week-old male infant

CC: Fever
The mother states that the infant has a fever. His rectal temperature is 101.9°F (38.8°C). The infant was seen by his Pediatrician 6 days ago, and received his Hepatitis B vaccine. He has been having a cold and oral thrush.

Disposition: The mother is advised that the infant must be checked now. She should take the neonate to ED to be examined. The 6-week-old infant with a fever should be checked immediately. Given the time that has elapsed since the immunization, the fever is most likely not related to the immunization. This child needs a septic work-up due to his young age.

## CASE #258

SPRING                                                                          TIME: 7:10AM

A nine-year-old male child

CC: Cough & history of asthma
The child has been coughing a great deal and has a history of asthma. His mother asks if she can start the asthma medicine.
Disposition: The mother is advised to start the asthma treatment (albuterol) immediately and repeat the albuterol in 20 minutes if he is still coughing a great deal. She may even repeat it again in 20 minutes and if he is getting better then she should continue every 4 hours and later every 6 hours as instructed. If there is any distress or no response to the albuterol at all, then he is to be seen at the ED. Otherwise, he can follow-up later at the clinic.

## CASE #259

SPRING                                                                          TIME: 7:48AM

A four-month-old male infant

CC: Rash
The infant has a rash all over the face, neck, and body that started today. Also, he has been cranky. He has been having a slight fever for the past two days.
Disposition: The mother is advised to have the infant examined today. A 4-month old fussy infant with a fever should be examined.

## CASE #260

SPRING                                                                          TIME: 5:10PM

An eleven-month-old male infant

CC: Fever & vomiting

The infant started vomiting yesterday. There was no bile and no blood in the vomitus. He has a fever today; his temperature taken from the axilla is 100.0°F (37.7°C). His bowel movement was normal yesterday and he has had no bowel movement today. His mother states she tried to give him clear fluid but he vomits and can not keep the fluid down.

Disposition: The mother is advised to start Pedialyte little by little (5mL each minute x 12 minutes), and observe. If he cannot retain the Pedialyte; then have him checked at the ED tonight. Otherwise, if he can hold the Pedialyte down; he may be checked tomorrow morning.


## CASE #261

LATE SPRING                                                    TIME: 8:23PM

A seven-year-old female child

CC: Diarrhea

The child has diarrhea that started today. She has not had any fever and there has been no vomiting. There is neither blood nor mucus in stool. There have been no recent antibiotics given and no recent travel.

Disposition: The mother is advised to give her Pedialyte and clear fluid (Gatorade, ginger ale) and to offer her foods like white rice, saltine or graham crackers, applesauce, banana and plain yogurt. The mother is to avoid offering the child milk and dairy products for a few days and to observe. The child is to be checked if the condition persists, if there is blood in the stool, or if the child is not urinating well (at least once every 6-8 hours).


## CASE #262

LATE SPRING                                                    TIME: 9:05PM

A two-month-old male infant

CC: Constipation

The infant has not had any bowel movements for 9-10 hours. He usually had been having two to three bowel movements per day. His mother states she started to feed him rice cereal in the bottle and that his formula also has been changed prior to his constipation.

Disposition: The mother is advised to offer the baby small amounts of juices like prune or pear juice diluted with water (one ounce of juice mixed with 3-4 oz. of water) and to stop the cereal. The infant has an appointment tomorrow morning to be checked and should keep this appointment.

## Case #263

A five-year-old female child

CC: Fever

The child, who attends preschool, currently has a fever of 103.3°F (39.6°C). She was seen by her pediatrician today and has been told that she has Strep Throat and she is on Penicillin, she was given one dose so far.

Disposition: The mother is advised to continue the Penicillin as instructed and give her Children's Tylenol (160mg/5mL, two teaspoons every 4-6 hours) or Motrin (100mg/5mL, 2 teaspoons every 6 to 8 hours) for the fever and fluid (water, juice, soup) and to observe. The child is to be reevaluated if she is not responding to the treatment in one or two days (one should give antibiotics 2-3 days to show an effect). In addition, it is recommended to get a new toothbrush for the child to use after the 5th day of the 10-day antibiotic course.

## Case #264

A 22-month-old female toddler

CC: Fever

The child started to have a fever at 12:00AM, her temperature is 103.0°F (39.4°C). Infants' Tylenol 160mg was given at 12:00AM and her mother just gave her 80mg of Children's Motrin as well. She has no vomiting. She drinks fluid well.

Disposition: Her mother is advised to put a cold compress on her forehead and under her arms to help bring her temperature down and to have her checked early this morning (later today), if the fever persists.

A child 2-year-old and younger with a fever ≥102.2F (39.0C) should be checked to rule out serious bacterial infections.

## Case #265

A ten-month-old male infant

CC: Diarrhea & vomiting

The infant has non-bloody, non-mucoid diarrhea, non-bloody, non- bilious vomiting and a fever. The mother has given him Pedialyte and Tylenol but the baby continues to have a fever, vomiting and diarrhea. He is urinating well.

Disposition: The mother is advised to have the infant checked today.

A 10-month-old infant with on-going diarrhea, vomiting and fever despite trial of the oral rehydration fluid and Tylenol, should be examined and treated. The mother should offer him Pedialyte in small amounts (5mL every minute x 12 minutes), and take him to be checked.

## CASE #266

A two-year-old male toddler

CC: Fever

The child started to have a fever today. He has no vomiting and no other problem. Tylenol was given for his fever but he continues to have a fever; his temperature is 102.0°F (38.8°C). He is drinking fluid well and urinating well.

Disposition: The mother is advised to give him Children's Motrin (100mg/5mL, 6mL every 6 to 8 hours) for fever and to observe him. If he is fine and playful, then the mother can wait and take him to be checked tomorrow.

## CASE #267

A three-month-old female infant

CC: Cold symptoms & cough

The infant has had cold symptoms and a cough since last night. She has no fever but her mother gave her 40mg of Infants' Tylenol today.

She is feeding well and urinating as usual.

Disposition: The mother is advised to use Normal Saline nose drops in her nostrils (1-2 drops into the nostrils, three or four times per day), a humidifier around the baby, and to observe her. If the cold persists or if she were to have a fever (rectal temperature of ≥100.4°F [38.0°C]) then she is to be examined.

## Case #268

A three-year-old female child

CC: Cold symptoms & fever
The child has been having cold symptoms for 4 days. She started to have a fever today. Her temperature is 102.0°F (38.8°C); no Tylenol has been given yet.
Disposition: The mother is advised to give her one teaspoon of Children's Tylenol (160mg/5mL) and to offer her more fluid (water, juice, soup) to drink, and to observe. If her temperature comes down and she is getting better, then the mother may wait and have the child checked tomorrow. If she continues to have a high fever despite the Tylenol, then the mother should take her to be examined at the ED tonight.

## Case #269

A four-year-old female child

CC: Abdominal pain
The child complains of abdominal pain. She has had no vomiting, and no fever. She complained of abdominal pain 2 days ago, which subsided. Her bowel movements are normal. Currently after she had corn and some other foods, she soon after started complaining of abdominal pain again.
Disposition: I recommended that the mother give her clear fluid (Pedialyte, ginger ale) and give her 0.6 mL of Infants' Mylicon drops (simethicone) and observe. She may be checked tomorrow.
Infants' Mylicon drops is an anti-flatulent. It is simethicone 20mg/0.3mL liquid and is alcohol free. Children above 2 years of age may have 0.6 mL after meals and at bed time as needed; a maximum of 12 doses may be given per day.

## Case #270

A 20-month-old female toddler

CC: Diaper rash
The child has a severe diaper rash since about 6 days ago. The mother has been

applying A& D ointment and another kind of soothing ointment but the rash is not getting better.

Disposition: The mother is advised to get Mycostatin ointment (antifungal) to apply on the diaper rash twice per day or to use cornstarch powder (not talc) tonight and have the toddler examined tomorrow.

The diaper rash which is not responding to the regular soothing ointments is most likely due to Candida species (yeast) infection. Topical Mycostatin ointment (Nystatin 100,000 units/g) 2-4 times per day will be an effective treatment.

## Case #271

Early summer                                              Time: 9:12PM

A six-month-old male infant

CC: Rash

The mother states that the infant has had a rash on his face and some parts of his body since yesterday. He has neither fever nor vomiting and his bowel movements have been normal.

Disposition: The mother is advised that if the infant has been hot/ sweating, then she is to bathe him more often and pat him dry and then apply cornstarch (not talc) and avoid letting him get too warm. Check to see that clothing and blankets are made of 100% cotton. The mother is also advised about the possibility of an allergic rash (she is asked if the rash might be related to a new food or drink that was just introduced to his diet, or a new soap or detergent that is to be avoided). If the rash appears to be bothering the child, the mother may use Calamine lotion on the rash and observe. She may have him checked in the clinic in the morning if she wants. If fever ≥102.2°F (39.0°C) should occur, then the child should be checked sooner.

## Case #272

Early summer                                              Time: 9:25PM

A 27-day-old female neonate

CC: Crying

The mother states that the baby has been crying after her feeding this evening. The mother believes that the crying after feeding may be because the baby wants to move her bowels but cannot. She has had a normal bowel movement today, and she has had no vomiting. She is feeding well and urinating as usual. She is not crying now.

Disposition: The mother is advised regarding gastro-esophageal reflux, and infantile colic and to avoid over feeding the baby. She is to have him checked if the condition persists.

## CASE #273

SUMMER                                                      TIME: 10:19PM

A one-year-old male infant

CC: Question about hepatitis

The mother is concern about contracting hepatitis since she just found out that her own father had hepatitis. The child also has a cold and cough and has an appointment to be checked tomorrow.

Disposition: The mother is advised regarding the types of hepatitis and the transmission of the different types of hepatitis and the immunizations against hepatitis B and hepatitis A. She should obtain information about her father's hepatitis and keep the baby's appointment at the clinic.

Hepatitis A virus is transmitted via contaminated foods. The household contacts of a person who has hepatitis A should receive prophylactic Immunoglobulin (IG, 0.02mL/kg body weight to be given if the exposure is less than two weeks) and there is a hepatitis A vaccine (for children 12 months and older) given in 2 doses, 6 months apart.

Hepatitis B and C are contracted through blood and body fluids contamination, and hepatitis B is transmitted vertically to the newborn infant from the affected mother. Hence the exposure to blood and body fluids should be avoided and the newborn infants should receive hepatitis B immunization soon after birth. If the mother is positive for hepatitis B surface antigen, the newborn infant should receive hepatitis B immunoglobulin as well, to be protected.

Hepatitis B immunizations are given in a 3-dose series. The second dose of hepatitis B is given one month after the first dose and the 3rd dose given 4-5 months after the 2nd dose. Hepatitis B immunizations should be done routinely; the mother should ensure the infant has received all his hepatitis B immunizations as well as other immunizations. There are other types of hepatitis like autoimmune hepatitis and hepatitis related to alcohol, drugs and some other viruses.

## CASE #274

SUMMER                                                      TIME: 10:15AM

A three-year-old male child

CC: Nausea

The mother states that the child had food poisoning a few days ago. He was hospitalized for 2-3 days and was discharged. He does not want to eat and wants to vomit after eating.

Disposition: His mother is advised to give him just clear fluid (white grape juice, flat ginger ale and Pedialyte), and to observe. After he can tolerate the fluid she may then try soft foods (applesauce, pudding and Jell-O) and then gradually regular foods.

## CASE #275

SUMMER                                                        TIME: 11:41AM

A 13-month-old male infant

Cc: Runny nose & eye congestion

The child has a runny nose, eye congestion, no fever, and he has been having loose bowel movements.

Disposition: The mother is advised regarding the use of Normal Saline nose drops (use 1-2 drops into the nostrils, three or four times per day) and fluid (Pedialyte, white grape juice and flat ginger ale) and to offer him foods like soft and well-cooked white rice, applesauce, banana, and plain yogurt. She may have him checked tomorrow. Enterovirus infections mostly occur during the summer time. Some are associated with nonspecific fever, coryza, eye congestion and loose bowel movement.

## CASE #276

SUMMER                                                        TIME: 1:02PM

A seven-month-old female infant

CC: Prefers drinking juice

The mother states that the infant is not drinking as much formula as she had been drinking before, but she is taking other fluid like juice. She has no other problem.

Disposition: The mother is advised to avoid offering her sweet fluid and juice and offer just her formula, and observe. She can also have 4-6 oz. of water each day, especially if it is hot outdoors.

## Case #277

Time: 1:20PM

A 20-year-old female adolescent

CC: Vaginal pruritis

The adolescent complains of vaginal itching. She had a pelvic examination 2 weeks ago, and received an injection of Depo- Provera (progestin 150mg, an IM injection). She is on Monistat vaginal cream.

Disposition: She is advised on the proper use of the Monistat and get in touch with the clinic to obtain her culture and wet mount results, and to be reexamined if required. It is possible that she may need oral medication, specifically Diflucan (an azole antifungal, fluconazole 150mg tablet), and to take one tablet once, if the wet mount reveals candida.

Beside candidiasis (yeast infection), trichomoniasis can also cause vulvovaginal pruritis and is associated with a malodorous frothy discharge and motile trichomonas that can be seen on the microscopic exams of vaginal discharge. The treatment for trichomoniasis is Metronidazole 2g in a single dose or 500mg twice daily for 7 days.

## Case #278

Summer                                                      Time: 3:43AM

A 19-month-old male toddler

CC: High fever & crankiness

The child has been crying excessively and has a fever. His temperature is 103.0°F (39.4°C). He was seen at an ED a few hours ago. The mother has been told that he has an ear infection. Children's Motrin and Amoxicillin were just given but he continues to be cranky, and he is crying and refusing to drink.

Disposition: The mother is advised on the proper dose of the Motrin. If it has been given at the correct dose and he is still crying inconsolably, and he is not feeling any better and still has a high fever, then he should be reexamined. Alternatively, a dose of Tylenol can also be given to see if that helps bring the high fever down and makes him feel better. For the fever and pain, he can have Children's Motrin 120mg every 6-8 hours, and Infants' Tylenol 120mg may also be given every 4-6 hours. They can also try to bring his temperature down with tepid sponging, continue to give proper doses of Amoxicillin as instructed, and to offer him fluids to drink. The Amoxicillin will take a couple of days to show an effect. In the meantime, the Motrin and Tylenol should be used for pain, however if he continues to be very cranky (inconsolable) and have a high fever despite these measures, then he may be taken back to the ED as there is a concern for possible meningitis.

## Case #279

SUMMER                                                      Time: 7:17AM

An 18-year-old female adolescent

CC: Flatulence

The adolescent girl complains of stomachache and gas. She had hardened bread yesterday and thinks that produced gas in her abdomen and it appears that the pain has now transferred to her chest. She now thinks that perhaps the hard bread may be stuck in her chest and feels tightness. She is also an asthmatic.

Disposition: Her chest tightness most likely is related to her asthma. She is advised to start to take her asthma medicine (albuterol metered dose inhaler) via the spacer, 2 puffs every 4 hours for a few days and when she is getting better, then she may use it every 6 hours and continue using it until she has no cough at all. She should also drink some fluid (water, juice, soup and ginger ale) and observe. She may be checked if the condition persists.

For the gas, she can use anti-flatulent medicine like simethicone 40mg after meals.

## Case #280

SUMMER                                                      Time: 5:00PM

A one-year-old female infant

CC: Insect bite

The child has an insect bite. The telephone number given by her mother to the answering service was not working and was disconnected; therefore, I could not get in touch with her to advise her. In the summer time, we receive some calls regarding the insect bites; use of Calamine lotion on the bite, preventive measures like avoiding taking the child out in the dusk, using safe insect repellents, and wearing long sleeves and long pants are suggested. We also determine if secondary infections may be taking place.

## Case #281

SUMMER                                                      Time: 5: 44PM

A one-year-old male infant

CC: Refusing to drink Pediasure

The mother states that the child is refusing to drink, but he is eating well and has been urinating well. He has no fever and no other problem. He is on Pediasure and he likes to eat baby food.

Disposition: His mother is reassured and advised to offer him small amount of water and fluid frequently and observe.

## CASE #282
SUMMER                                                                TIME: 7:51PM

A 15-month-old female toddler

CC: Request for more antibiotics

The child had a fever for 2-3 days. They were just in Canada. She was seen by a physician in Canada and received Children's Tylenol and an antibiotic and was told that the child had an infection of the throat. The mother states the child is doing well now but she needs another prescription for antibiotics because the Canadian prescription was not accepted in the United States.

Disposition: The mother is advised to make sure the child is fine; if she is not developing any higher fevers and is drinking well, then she can be observed this evening. I recommended that the mother keep the toddler's clinic appointment in the morning and that she may obtain a new prescription at that time.

## CASE #283
SUMMER                                                                TIME: 8:24PM

A one-month-old male infant

CC: Colic

The infant drinks breastmilk and has developed colic (periods of crying but fine in between). He has no other problem. The baby is feeding well. He has neither fever nor vomiting.

Disposition: His mother is advised to refrain from eating gas producing foods (onion, radishes, and beans) and to avoid drinking cow's milk (but she is to be sure to drink enough fluid). Mother is also advised to cuddle the baby and observe to see that he is consolable. The mother is asked to have him checked at the clinic if the symptoms persist despite these measures. If he were to have a fever or fail to be consoled, then he may need to be checked sooner.

## Case #284

A four-year-old male child

CC: Streptococcal throat infection & refusing to drink
The child was seen by a physician and received a penicillin injection because of Strep throat. He complains of mouth pain and refuses to drink.
Disposition: The mother is advised to give him mild liquids and soft foods in small amounts and to rinse his mouth with plain water after he eats and observe. She may also give him a dose of Children's Tylenol or Children's Motrin for pain.

## Case #285

Summer                                                   Time: 9:06PM

An eleven-week-old male infant

CC: Cold symptoms & spitting up
The infant has been having a cold and cough for 2 days.
He has no fever. He is exclusively breastfed and spits up after each feeding.
Disposition: The mother is advised to use Normal Saline nose drops (1-2 drops into the nostrils, three or four times per day) and a humidifier in the room. The mother is asked to feed the baby for a shorter time but more frequently at the breast and to observe. If there is no fever, he may be checked tomorrow.

## Case #286

Summer                                                   Time: 5:09PM

A two-month-old female infant

CC: Oral thrush
The infant has whitish spots on her tongue and inside her lips for 2 days. The infant is otherwise doing well.
Disposition: The mother is advised that a medication will be ordered to her pharmacy for the baby. The mother is to get the medicine from the pharmacy and use one

milliliter into both sides of the infant's mouth four times per day until the whitish spots in the mouth clear up completely. Alternatively, she may paint the spots with the medicine using a Q-tip, four times daily. She should continue to use the medicine for 2-3 days more after the clearance of the whitish spots. The medication Nystatin 100,000 units per milliliter oral suspension is ordered via phone, and is to be picked up by the mother. The baby's pacifiers should be sterilized.

The infant has oral thrush and needs an antifungal medication (Nystatin). The medication should be used on the whitish spots on the mucous membrane of the mouth and will be swallowed by the infant. The medication will have both topical and systemic effects.

If the mother is breastfeeding, then she may also apply the medication to her nipples, also four times daily, also for three days beyond the resolution of symptoms.

## CASE #287

SUMMER                                                    TIME: 5:23PM

A one-month-old male neonate

CC: Crying
The infant had excessive crying.
The mother did not respond to the answering service return call. The answering service left a message for her but, she had probably taken the infant to the ED.

## CASE #288

SUMMER                                                    TIME: 7:10PM

A three-week-old female neonate

CC: Diarrhea
The baby has had very loose and watery stool about four times today. She has no other problem.
Disposition: The mother is advised that if the stools are of a large volume, then she should start Pedialyte for a few feedings then offer the baby Lactose-free formula and observe. The baby is to be checked if the condition persists.

## CASE #289

SUMMER                                                    TIME: 7:58PM

A two-year-old male toddler

CC: Fever & poor appetite
The child has a fever; his temperature is 102.0°F (38.8°C) and he has lost his appetite. He vomited once last night and his temperature was 104.0°F (40.0°C), Motrin was given.
Disposition: The mother is advised to give him Children's Motrin (100 mg/5 mL, 6 mL every 6 to 8 hours) or Children's Tylenol (160 mg/5mL, one teaspoon every 4-6 hours) for his fever and to offer him more fluid (water, juice, soup, ginger ale) and observe. If the high fever persists despite these measures, then he is to be checked tonight. Otherwise, he may be seen tomorrow morning.

## Case #290
SUMMER                                                    TIME: 7:10AM

A one-year-old female infant

CC: Cold symptoms
The infant has been having cold symptoms for two days. She has no fever. She is feeding well.
Disposition: The mother is advised to use Normal Saline nose drops in the baby's nostrils, 3-4 times per day and offer her more fluid to drink and observe. She may also use a humidifier.
Rhinovirus infections are the most common cause of cold symptoms. While these infections occur throughout the year, the peak prevalence is in autumn and spring.

## Case #291
LATE SUMMER                                               TIME: 7:30PM

A 16-month-old male toddler

CC: Mosquito bites
The child has an itchy skin lesion for 2 days. His mother thought it was a mosquito bite, but he appears to be getting more lesions. He has no fever and no other problems.
Disposition: The mother is advised to use Calamine lotion on the lesions and observe. If there are no improvements, then the child may be checked tomorrow if required.
Calamine lotion is a skin protectant. It soothes and protects the skin. Hydrocortisone 1% cream, a low potency steroid also can help with itch, it may be used when we are

sure there is no sign of a skin infection, as infections can be made worse as a result.

## Case# 292

A three-month-old female infant

CC: Cold symptoms & sneezing
The infant has had a cold and has been sneezing for 2-3 days. She has no fever and no other problem. She is taking the formula well.
Disposition: The mother is advised to use Normal Saline nose drops (1-2 drops into the nostrils, 3-4 times per day) and observe. She is to be examined if the cold is not getting better or she has any fever.

## Case #293

A five-month-old male infant

CC: Diarrhea
The infant has had diarrhea for 2-3 days. He has no fever and no vomiting. He urinates well; there is neither blood nor mucus in his stool.
Disposition: The mother is advised to give him Pedialyte and clear fluid (white grape juice). When he is getting better, she may then start rice cereal and Lactose-free formula and observe. He is to be checked if the condition persists.

## Case #294

A four-month-old female infant

CC: Runny nose
The father states that the baby has been having a runny nose for one or two days. He thinks that the baby probably has a slight fever. His temperature taken rectally is 99.0°F (37.2°C).
Disposition: The father is advised that a rectal temperature below 100.4°F (38.0°C) is considered normal. Use of Normal Saline nose drops (1-2 drops into the nostrils, 3-4 times per day) and Infants' Tylenol 40mg every 4-6 hours for fever, is advised and the

baby is to be observed. If there is a fever ≥102.2°F (39.0°C), then the baby should be checked.

## Case #295

A one-month-old female neonate

CC: Constipation
The mother states that the baby has been constipated for 2-3 days.
Her abdomen appears to be hard and she is very cranky.
Disposition: The mother is advised to take the baby to the ED to be checked. When a neonate has constipation associated with a hardened abdomen and is being very cranky, the infant must be checked.

## Case #296

A four-year-old male child

CC: Exacerbation of asthma
The child is an asthmatic and he started wheezing early this morning. The asthma medicine (albuterol) was given via the nebulizer about one hour ago, but he continues to have wheezing.
Disposition: The mother is advised to use the albuterol solution for inhalation via the nebulizer again and to then repeat the treatment in 20 minutes if there is still any wheezing. If the wheezing is improving after these measures, then she may continue the albuterol via the nebulizer every four to six hours and observe. She is to have him checked if the child is in any distress (having retractions, flaring the nasal alae, and using the abdominal muscles to breathe) or if not responding to albuterol.

## Case #297

A one-month-old female neonate

CC: Constipation
The baby has been constipated. She was examined and received advice previously. She

has no vomiting and her abdomen looks fine and is soft with no distension.

Disposition: The mother is advised regarding the baby's diet. She may offer her boiled then cooled water to drink and she may also take a gentle rectal temperature with small amount of Vaseline on the tip of the thermometer, and observe. Also, she may bicycle the legs and massage the abdomen in a clockwise fashion.

## CASE #298

LATE SUMMER                                                         TIME: 5:00PM

A two-month-old male infant

CC: Diarrhea

The infant has been having diarrhea for one or two days. He has been having four bowel movements per day. His stool has been very loose and sometimes there is a large amount. There has been neither blood nor mucus in the stool. He has no fever and no vomiting. He urinates well and is feeding well.

Disposition: The mother is advised to start Pedialyte instead of formula for a few feedings and then to start a Lactose-free formula and observe. He has an appointment to be checked tomorrow and if he continues to urinate well, he may wait until then to be seen.

## CASE #299

LATE SUMMER                                                         TIME: 5:15PM

A two-year-old male toddler

CC: Fever & stomachache

The child has a fever; his temperature is 101.0°F (38.3°C) and he has been complaining of a stomachache since about one hour ago. He has no vomiting. Children's Motrin was given for his fever.

Disposition: The mother is advised to give him clear fluid (Pedialyte, flat ginger ale) and observe. If he continues to have the pain, then he may need to be checked.

## CASE #300

LATE SUMMER                                                         TIME: 5:45 PM

A six-year-old male child

CC: Round lesions on the face and neck

The child has been having round lesions on his face and neck for a few days. His mother has been using hydrocortisone cream on the lesions which helps, but the lesions reappear again.

Disposition: The mother is advised to call and make an appointment tomorrow to be checked and receive the proper treatment.

The round lesions could be nummular atopic dermatitis (allergic dry skin) or tinea facialis or tinea corporis (fungal).

A solitary round lesion, sometimes multiple, could be the site of a recent tick bite and early manifestation of lyme disease. This lesion is called erythema migrans and usually gets larger. It starts as a small red flat or raised lesion and then forms a large annular (ring-shaped) lesion. The lesions of lyme disease are usually accompanied by fever and malaise, myalgia and arthralgia.

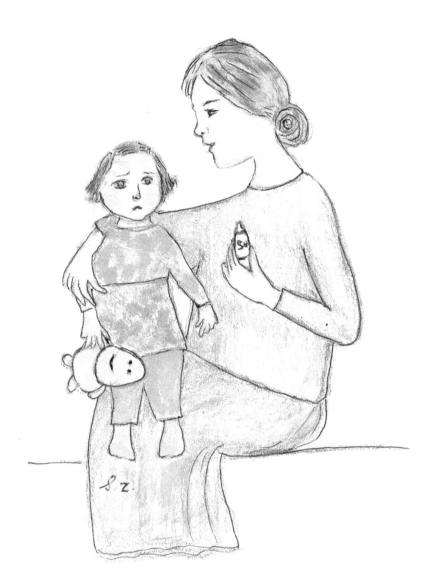

A Toddler with Cold

# Chapter Seven

⚬⚬⚬

## Case #301

Late summer                                          Time: 9:04PM

A two-year-old male toddler

CC: Rash

The child has a rash on some parts of his face and body. The mother first noticed the rash when he woke up this morning. There are two bumps on his forehead, one on his cheek and one on his thigh. He has no fever. The lesions are itchy.

Disposition: The mother is advised to use Calamine lotion on the bumps, three or four times per day, to take care of the skin to prevent infection, and to observe.

The child appears to have insect bites, since the skin lesions are mostly on the exposed areas. Discrete itchy lesions could also herald chickenpox (VZV), now a vaccine-preventable illness.

## Case #302

Late summer                                          Time: 7:25AM

A six-year-old male child

CC: Fever, headache, & stomachache

The child has been having a fever for two or three days. He complains of a headache and a stomachache.

Disposition: His mother is advised to give him Children's Tylenol (160mg/5mL, 2 teaspoons every 4-6 hours) or Children's Motrin (100mg/5mL, 2 teaspoons every 6-8 hours) for his fever, and to offer him more fluid (juice, soup, ginger ale) to drink. The mother is asked to call and make an appointment and have him examined today at the clinic. Streptococcal pharyngitis occurs at all ages but is most common in school-aged children. Group A Streptococcal infection is often associated with headache and stomachache in addition to a sore throat.

## CASE #303
EARLY AUTUMN                                                    TIME: 5:20PM

A five-month-old male infant

CC: Noisy breathing
The infant had noisy breathing today. He was seen by a physician today and medicine was prescribed by phone to a pharmacy, but the mother could not obtain it. She wants to obtain the medication at a different pharmacy, and wants the medicine to be called in. Disposition: The mother is advised to find the name of the medicine that was prescribed by calling and asking the original pharmacy, as the infant has no history of wheezing nor asthma in the past.
If the noisy breathing is from nasal congestion, then Normal Saline nose drops will be ordered and if the noise is coming from his chest and the infant is wheezing, then he needs an albuterol MDI and a spacer.

## CASE #304
EARLY AUTUMN                                                    TIME: 5:53PM

A one-month-old male neonate

CC: Cough & cold symptoms
The mother states that the baby has a cough and cold symptoms that started today. He has no fever, no vomiting, and no wheezing. He is taking the formula well, and is urinating well.
Disposition: The mother is advised to use Normal saline nose drops (1-2 drops into the nostrils, three or four times per day), to put a humidifier in the room around the baby, and to observe. She may have the baby checked tomorrow in the clinic, since he is just one-month-old.

## Case #305

An eight-month-old male infant

CC: Cold symptoms

The mother states that the infant has had a cold and watery eyes and nose for two days. He has neither fever nor vomiting, he has been slightly cranky but he is taking formula well, and urinating adequately.

Disposition: The mother is advised to offer him fluid (white grape juice, apple juice, broth and formula or breast milk) and use Normal Saline nose drops (1-2 drops into the nostrils, 3-4 times per day), and observe. She may have him checked tomorrow, if she is concerned that he is worsening or not improving, or if there is a fever ≥102.2°F (39.0°C).

## Case #306

A three-year-old male child

CC: Bloody diarrhea

The mother states that the child developed diarrhea for one hour. He had a watery stool with blood and mucus in it. He has neither fever nor vomiting.

Disposition: The mother is advised to give him Pedialyte and clear fluid (white grape juice, flat ginger ale) and to have him examined first thing this morning. The child needs to have a test for stool culture and a stool test for ova and parasite and perhaps a blood test for complete blood count (CBC) and electrolytes.

## Case #307

A 19-year-old female adolescent

CC: Swollen tonsils

The adolescent had swollen tonsils and needed advice. I called her several times to speak with her but her line was busy. She should gargle with warm water with pinch of salt added to it. If she has sore throat, then she is to be checked tomorrow and have a throat culture taken.

# Case #308

Autumn                                                    Time: 6:45PM

A four-year-old female child

CC: Cold & earache
The child has been having a cold for a few days. She was seen at the clinic and has been told that she had a viral infection. She has developed an earache today. Children's ibuprofen (100mg/5mL) was given.
Disposition: The father is advised that the child needs to be reexamined and may need to receive an antibiotic if she has signs of ear infection.

# Case #309

Autumn                                                    Time: 7:30PM

A three-year-old male toddler

CC: Fever & asthma
The child has a history of bronchial asthma. He was seen at a Pediatric clinic two days ago, and received Tylenol and asthma medicine via a nebulizer. The child now has continued fevers; his temperature is 103.0°F (39.4°C) currently.
Disposition: His mother is advised to give him Children's Motrin (100mg/5mL, one and one-half teaspoons every 6-8 hours for fever) and to keep using the asthma medication (albuterol) as instructed for his cough. She is to offer him fluid (juice, soup, ginger ale) to drink and observe. The mother is also asked to have him reexamined the next day if a fever ≥102.2°F (39.0°C) persists overnight. If his cough is worsening or he is having any difficulty breathing, then he may be examined in the ED if needed tonight.

# Case #310

Autumn                                                    Time: 9:55PM

A six-year-old female child

CC: Dog bite
The child had been bitten by a dog 2-3 days ago. She has a skin abrasion and a shallow wound to the back of her right hand. She has not been seen for this ailment.
Disposition: The mother is advised to take the child to be checked and receive a

Tetanus shot if required (if the child is not up to date for her DTaP immunization) and a Rabies vaccine if the dog was not vaccinated. Also, she needs to receive oral antibiotics for the bite to prevent infection since pasteurella species is found in the oral flora of 25-50% of dogs and this pathogen causes skin and connective tissue infection (cellulitis). The drug of choice for the treatment of a suspected polymicrobial dog bite is oral amoxicillin-clavulanate (Augmentin).

## Case #311

Autumn                                                        Time: 10:55PM

A four-month-old female infant

CC: Crying in the evening
The father states the baby has been crying this evening. She has neither fever nor vomiting; her bowel movement is normal and her abdomen appears fine. She takes the formula well.
Disposition: The father is advised to cuddle the baby and to observe. The father is to take the baby to be checked if she continues to be cranky. Sometimes the infants cry in the evening, but if it is excessive and the baby is not consolable then the infant should be examined.

## Case #312

Autumn                                                        Time: 7:55AM

A six-week-old male infant

CC: Constipation
The baby has had constipation since yesterday. He has been cranky today. His temperature is 100.2°F (37.8°C). He has no vomiting; he takes the formula well and urinates well.
Disposition: The mother is advised to offer him boiled then cooled water to drink and to have him checked today.

## Case #313

Autumn                                                        Time: 7:45AM

An eleven-month-old female infant

CC: Diarrhea

The infant has been having diarrhea since yesterday. She has neither fever nor has she been vomiting. She takes the formula well, and urinates adequately. There is no blood and no mucus in the stool.

Disposition: The mother is advised to start Pedialyte for a few feedings. When her diarrhea is better, she is then to give her Lactose-free formula. Later, she can put her on a diet for those with diarrhea (rice cereal, applesauce, banana, plain yogurt), and continue Lactose-free formula, fluid, and observe. She is to have her examined if the condition persists, if there is blood in stool, if there is any abdominal pain, or if the baby is not urinating at least once every 6-8 hours.

## CASE #314

AUTUMN                                                                    TIME: 8:50AM

A four-year-old female child

CC: Child with sickle cell disease needing a medication refill
The child has sickle cell disease and is on prophylactic penicillin and has run out of the medicine.

Disposition: The mother is advised to go to the pharmacy to pick up the medication and the medicine will be ordered by phone.

Children with sickle cell disease should receive prophylactic penicillin at least up to the age of 5. They receive 125mg of oral penicillin twice per day up to 3 years of age and then 250mg of oral penicillin twice per day thereafter. The mother is advised to keep the scheduled follow-up appointment.

## CASE #315

AUTUMN                                                                   TIME: 11:26AM

A five-year-old child

CC: A call from a pharmacy
The call is from a pharmacy regarding a prescription for a five-year-old child. The medication is Amoxicillin 400 mg per 5 mL and the dose of the medicine is 2 teaspoons two times per day for one month. The pharmacist states that the medicine is a high dose and too long of a duration for a 5-year-old child and he thinks it might be a mistake. It is the weekend.

Disposition: I knew the pediatrician who wrote the prescription. She is a physician for the children with special needs and high-risk cases. I advised that they begin giving the medication at 1 teaspoon or 400 mg twice per day, and that they get in touch with the prescribing physician for confirmation and clarification on Monday.

## Case #316

An 18-month-old female toddler

CC: Head injury
The caregiver states that the child hit her head on the edge of the wall and that she cried immediately; she has had no loss of consciousness, but she does have a lump on the forehead.
Disposition: The caregiver is advised to apply an ice pack wrapped in a towel to the toddler's forehead for 15 minutes every hour, and to observe. If the child is irritable, vomiting, or acting out of the ordinary she may be checked.

## Case #317

A two-year-old male child

CC: Gagging & sometimes vomiting
The mother states that the child gags and vomits sometimes, for the past three or four days. He has neither fever nor any other problem and he looks fine. He had Strep Throat two weeks ago, and received a penicillin injection.
Disposition: The mother is advised to offer him fluid (white grape juice, Pedialyte, flat ginger ale) and to have him checked tomorrow if the condition were to persist.

## Case #318

A one-month-old female neonate

CC: Cough & congestion
The baby has had a cough and congestion today. She has neither fever nor vomiting; she is taking the formula well.
Disposition: The mother is advised to use Normal Saline nose drops (1-2 drops into

the nostrils, three or four times per day), put on a humidifier in the room around the baby, and observe. She may have her checked tomorrow (weekend call). A neonate with cough should be checked.

## CASE #319

AUTUMN                                                          TIME: 2:10PM

A one-week-old male neonate

CC: Umbilical cord bleeding
The father states that the baby's umbilical cord is sloughing and has slight bleeding around it.
Disposition: The father is advised to clean the umbilical stump with rubbing alcohol and that he may cover it with a sterile gauze or a bandage and observe.

## CASE #320

AUTUMN                                                          TIME: 2:27PM

A ten-year-old male child

CC: Medication refill order
The child has a history of bronchial asthma and needs his asthma medicine, namely a Proventil MDI.
Disposition: The Pharmacy was called and the medication was ordered via phone to the pharmacy to be picked up by the parents.
The father is advised to keep his scheduled appointment for asthma follow-up.

## CASE #321

AUTUMN                                                          TIME: 2:53PM

A two-year-old female toddler

CC: Blood in stool
The child's mother states that she has noticed some blood in her child's stool when she was emptying the potty. She says the child is not constipated, and did not complain of any pain. She is otherwise fine.
Disposition: The mother is advised to observe and to have the child checked tomorrow. Polyps and cow's milk allergy are among the culprits of painless bloody stool.

# Case #322

A one-month-old female neonate

CC: Colic
The baby has colic and has been cranky periodically after feeding and passing gas.
Disposition: The mother is advised to cuddle and swaddle the baby and avoid over feeding her. She may try a Lactose-free formula and observe. If the baby is not consolable, then she is to be examined.

# Case #323

A nine-month-old male infant

CC: Cough & vomited phlegm
The infant has vomited phlegm. He has been having a cold, and has been coughing for 4-5 days; he has not had any fever.
Disposition: The mother is advised to offer the baby clear fluid (water, apple juice or white grape juice and broth) and to use Normal Saline nose drops 1-2 drops into his nostrils, 3-4 times per day to wash out the mucous membrane of his nasopharynx. She could also use a humidifier in the room, and observe. If the cold and cough are not getting better or if he were to develop a fever, then she is to have him examined.

# Case #324

An eleven-year-old female child

CC: Sickle cell disease & cough
The child has slight cough for 2 days; she has no fever. Her temperature is 98.5°F (36.9°C). The child is known to have sickle cell disease and is on prophylactic penicillin.
Disposition: The father is advised to keep the child well-hydrated. He is to give her enough fluid to drink and observe. She is to be checked in case of fever, or if not getting better.
Prophylactic Penicillin is used for the sickle cell disease patients at least up to 5 years of age. However, some physicians want to continue it beyond that period for more

protection against encapsulated pathogens. The child with sickle cell disease should be vaccinated with both series of pneumococcal conjugate vaccine, 13-valent (PCV13) before 2 years of age as well as the pneumococcal polysaccharide vaccine, 23-valent (PPSV23) at 24 months of age. A second dose of PPSV23 should be administered 5 years later. In cases where a child with sickle cell disease had received pneumococcal conjugate vaccine, 7-valent (PCV7), they should receive PCV13 later as supplement. In this case at 24 month of age the PCV13 should be given first, and PPSV23 should be given 8 weeks later.

## CASE #325

WINTER                                                              TIME: 8:53AM

A ten-year-old male child

CC: Earache & jaw ache
The child has an earache and jaw ache since yesterday. His mother has been giving him Motrin since yesterday but he still has this problem. He has not had any fever, but he has been taking Motrin 200mg every 6 hours.
Disposition: The mother is advised to take the child in to be examined today. The child with an earache should be examined and if there is a sign of ear infection on exam, then he or she is to receive proper antibiotics.

## CASE #326

WINTER                                                              TIME: 10:12AM

A six-month-old male infant

CC: Cough
The infant has had a slight cough for 2 days, and now has yellowish mucus from his nose. He has no fever and he is fine otherwise.
Disposition: The mother is advised to use Normal Saline nose drops (1-2 drops into the nostrils, three or four times per day for 5-7 days) to wash out the mucus and to offer the baby more fluid like diluted juice, and water in addition to his formula or breastmilk to drink. She could also use a humidifier around the infant and observe. If the infant were to develop a fever, or if the cold is not getting better after one week, then she should have the infant checked.

# CASE #327

WINTER                                              TIME: 11:00AM

An eleven-year-old female child

CC: Vomiting & abdominal cramps

The child has been vomiting and has been having abdominal cramps today. Her sibling also has the same problem. There is no blood, and no bile in the vomitus; she has had no fever. Her bowel movements had been normal yesterday.

Disposition: The mother is advised to offer her Pedialyte and clear fluid (Gatorade, ginger ale) in small amounts, and to make sure she can retain this and to observe. If the symptoms persist or intensify despite having clear fluids, then the mother may have her checked today. Since another sibling has the same problem, they both most likely have a viral illness.

# CASE #328

WINTER                                              TIME: 11:05AM

A nine-year-old female child

CC: Vomiting & abdominal cramps

The child has had vomiting and has been complaining of abdominal cramps, her sibling also has the same problem, no new foods or foods out of the home were taken. She has neither fever nor diarrhea; there is no blood nor bile in the vomitus.

Disposition: The mother is advised to give her Pedialyte and clear fluid like ginger ale and Gatorade and is to make sure that she can retain it. She may have her checked if the condition (vomiting and abdominal cramps) persists.

Rotavirus infections are more prevalent during the cooler seasons.

Adenovirus cause enteric infections and occur throughout the year.

Enterovirus infections may manifest gastrointestinal symptoms like diarrhea, vomiting and abdominal pain, and in temperate climates, occur mostly in the summer and fall.

# CASE #329

WINTER                                              TIME: 11:15AM

A two-year-old female toddler

CC: Cold symptoms

The child has had congestion and a runny nose. She has no fever and no history of asthma.

Disposition: The mother is advised to use Normal Saline nose drops into the child's nostrils 3-4 times per day for 3-5 days and to use a humidifier in the room. She may offer her fluid (juice, soup, ginger ale) and observe. If there is a fever or if the cold is lasting more than one week without signs of improvement, then she may have her checked.

## CASE #330
WINTER                                            TIME: 11:20AM

A five-year-old male child

CC: Croupy cough
The child has a barking cough; he has neither fever nor vomiting. He has history of croup in the past; he has no history of asthma.

Disposition: The mother is advised to use warm steam around him and to offer him warm fluid and observe. A cool mist humidifier may also be used. She may have him checked if he is in any distress or if he is worsening and not improving with these measures.

## CASE #331
WINTER                                            TIME: 2:10PM

A 20-month-old female toddler

CC: Antibiotic-associated diarrhea
The child has had diarrhea. She had an ear infection last week and had initially received Amoxicillin and then the antibiotic was changed to Augmentin. She developed diarrhea after taking the Augmentin. She was then seen by her physician and received an antibiotic by injection. She has continued to have diarrhea; she has neither vomiting nor fever. There is no blood nor mucus in the stool.

Disposition: The mother is advised to give her Pedialyte and clear fluid (flat ginger ale), to offer her foods like well-cooked white rice, applesauce, banana, plain yogurt, and to observe. If the condition persists and the child is not voiding every 6 to 8 hours, or if there is abdominal pain or blood in stool, then the mother should have the toddler seen at the hospital.

The prolonged use of antibiotic disrupts the normal intestinal florae and promotes the colonization of clostridium difficile; an anaerobic, gram positive bacillus organism and cause of infection.

C. difficile results in a diarrheal illness ranging from mild self-limited disease, to an explosive watery diarrhea with mucus and occult blood, and even to a more severe form known as Pseudomembranous colitis, that is associated with bacteremia and fever.

## Case #332

Time: 2:18PM

An 18-day-old male neonate

CC: Fever
The neonate has a temperature of 100.4°F (38.0°C) taken from axilla. The neonate had been in the neonatal intensive care unit.
Disposition: The mother is advised to see if the temperature is not related to over-wrapping the baby and very warm environment. She is to unbundle and retake the temperature in the rectum if possible. If the temperature is ≥100.4°F (38.0°C), then she is to take the baby to the hospital to be evaluated.

## Case #333

Winter                                                                    Time; 8:15PM

A 16-month-old female toddler

CC: Vomiting
The mother states that the child has been vomiting today. Her mother started Pedialyte for her but she vomited the Pedialyte. There is no blood nor bile in the vomitus. Her father also has the same problem.
Disposition: The mother is advised to give her Pedialyte in small amounts (sip by sip or with a spoon) and to observe. If she cannot retain the Pedialyte, then she is to be seen at hospital. Given that the father has the same symptoms, there is a high likelihood that the illness has a viral origin.

## Case #334

Winter                                                                    Time: 10:50PM

A two-year-old male toddler

CC: Poor appetite

The child has had a lack of an appetite for two days. He is not eating solid food but he is taking in juice and Pedialyte. He did have a fever for two days and he has no fever today; he has normal bowel movement, and is urinating well.

Disposition: The father is advised to give him fluids (juice, soup, ginger ale) and then to gradually give him soft foods and then regular food. He may give him multivitamin drops (Poly-Vi-Sol) 1.0mL daily and observe. The father is also advised to make an appointment for the toddler to be checked (2-year well visit) and have a complete blood count to make sure he is not anemic, since iron deficiency anemia can cause a poor appetite. Also, a blood test for screening for lead exposure (a lead level) is warranted at the 2-year well visit.


## CASE #335

WINTER                                                                TIME: 11:33PM

An eleven-day-old male neonate

CC: Bleeding from umbilical stump

The mother states that the baby's umbilical cord fell off last night; his umbilical stump was irritated by the diaper and has had some bleeding. He also has been feeding more frequently and vomited once today; he has no other problem.

Disposition: The mother is advised to clean the umbilical stump with rubbing alcohol and to then cover it with sterile gauze and observe. She is to make sure there is no discharge nor odor from the umbilical stump. She is to avoid feeding the baby frequently because it takes about 3-4 hours for the stomach to empty, and if the infant is fed atop of the previous feeding, the stomach may not have enough capacity, and so the infant will vomit.

During the beginning of the first month, because the newborn babies take smaller amount of formula or breastmilk, the newborn could be fed on demand but still not sooner than one, or preferably two hours. Holding the baby vertically after each feeding, burping, and the creation of an incline in the crib by placing a sheet or towel under the mattress (nothing in the crib) so that the baby's head is always elevated, also help to minimize the emesis.

If there is discharge or a foul odor from the umbilical stump or there is continued un-explained vomiting despite the recommended measures, then the neonate may be checked.


## CASE #336

WINTER                                                                TIME: 5:00AM

A three-month-old male infant

CC: Cough

The infant has had a cough. His mother states the baby bas been on albuterol for his cough, and when it is used he has no cough. There is no other problem.

Disposition: The mother is advised to continue to use the albuterol as instructed and observe. If there is any fever or other new symptoms, then she may have him checked. She should keep his appointment for bronchiolitis/asthma follow-up.


## Case #337
Winter                                                          Time: 5:10AM

A five-year-old female

CC: Fever

The child has a fever; her temperature is 104.0°F (40.0°C). Children's Tylenol has been given. She also has a slight cough and a headache. She has had no vomiting, but does have nausea.

Disposition: The grandmother is advised that if the temperature is not coming down with the use of antipyretics, then she should take the child to be checked. Children's Tylenol (160mg per 5mL), 2 teaspoons every 4-6 hours, and Children's Motrin (100mg per5mL), 2 teaspoons every 6-8 hours, may be given to control her fever. The grandmother is also advised to offer her fluid (water, juice, soup, ginger ale) and may wait to have her checked later today if she is tolerating these measures.


## Case #338
Winter                                                          Time: 8:24AM

A seven-year-old female child

CC: Cold & an earache

The child has a cold and has had pink eyes for a few days. She has been complaining about her ears hurting since yesterday. Today she is complaining about both ears and has a subjective fever.

Disposition: The mother is advised to take her to be examined.

As you notice the time of the call is in the morning and the child complaining of ear pain with probable fever is better off getting checked during the daytime by a physician. If they were to wait, the condition would likely only get worse and so it is better not to delay care. Also, patients and their families might wish to visit the ED at night given the severe pain that can result. However, ear infections are best seen and treated in the pediatrician's office or clinic.

## CASE #339
WINTER                                                    TIME: 9:25AM

A three-year-old male toddler

CC: Fever
The child has been having a fever for two days.
I called the telephone number provided by the answering service, but could not get in touch with the family. The three-year-old toddler with 2 days of fever was probably taken in to be checked per his mother's preference, rather than waiting for telephone advice.

## CASE #340
WINTER                                                    TIME: 9:30AM

A 20-month-old female toddler

CC: Foreign body exposure to the eyes
The mother state that a kind of oil-based perfume was splashed to the child's eyes accidentally.
Disposition: The mother is advised to use a great deal of water to wash the eyes and if the child has any complaints after this measure, then she is to be taken to the ED.

## CASE #341
WINTER                                                    TIME: 10:30AM

A nine-month-old male infant

CC: Vomiting & cold symptoms
The infant was seen at the ED yesterday and has been told he had a stomach virus, a cold, and an ear infection. He is supposed to be on Amoxicillin, but his mother states that she was not able to give him the Amoxicillin; she is just giving him the Pedialyte and he has not been vomiting anymore.
Disposition: The mother is advised that if the infant is having a fever and was diagnosed

by a physician as having an ear infection, then she should start the antibiotic as instructed and keep the appointment for follow-up.

## Case #342

A six-year-old female child

CC: Fever & vomiting

The mother states that the child has been having a fever for two days and has been vomiting today. Tylenol has been given. However, she continues to have a fever. She has vomited once today. There is no blood nor bile in the vomitus; she has had no diarrhea.

Disposition: The mother is advised to give her Children's Tylenol (160mg per 5 mL, 2 teaspoons every 4-6 hours) or Children's Motrin (100 mg per 5mL, 2 teaspoons every 6-8 hours) for fever and to offer her clear fluid (Pedialyte, ginger ale, Gatorade) since she has been vomiting. She may take her to be examined today, if she is not improving with these measures. Fever and vomiting may be the signs of a viral infection. However, several bacterial infections including urinary tract infections, pneumonias, ear infections and Strep pharyngitis also have fever and vomiting as symptoms. However, these will often have other accompanying symptoms.

## Case #343

A seven-month-old female infant

CC: Fever & pallor

The infant had a fever and she appears very pale. Her mother just gave her 130mg of Infants' Tylenol for fever. The baby has been congested and cranky.

Disposition: The mother is advised regarding the dose of Infants' Tylenol. The dose is weight dependent, 10-15mg/kg/dose. For a seven- month-old infant, 80mg of Infants' Tylenol may be given every 4-6 hours for a fever (a temperature ≥ 100.4ºF [38.0ºC]). She is to also offer the baby some fluid (juice, formula, water) and to take her in to be examined today.

## CASE #344

TIME: 1:47PM

An 18-month-old female toddler

CC: Finger injury

The child's finger was caught in between the door and its frame and is now slightly swollen. The mother had applied a cold compress on it and it appears to be getting better and she can move her finger.

Disposition: The mother is advised to use a small ice pack wrapped in a towel for 10-15 minutes every 30 minutes on the child's finger and to observe. She has an appointment to see her physician tomorrow, and so can wait until then to be checked if the child's pain is well-controlled.

## CASE #345

WINTER

TIME: 4:55PM

A four-month-old female infant

CC: Fever

The infant has a fever. Her axillary temperature is 101.0°F (38.3°C). Her mother and a sibling also have a fever.

Disposition: Her mother is advised to give the baby 40mg of Infants' Tylenol every 4-6 hours for a rectal temperature of ≥100.4°F (38.0°C), to offer her water to drink, and to observe. If the baby is fine (eating well, voiding normally, acting normally) and the fever is less than 102.2°F (39.0°C) (rectal temperature preferred), then the baby may be checked tomorrow. Otherwise, she may be taken to the ED to be examined tonight. As the mother and a sibling also have a fever; it appears that the fever may have a viral origin. However, if the fever is high, then the baby should be checked given her young age.

## CASE #346

WINTER

TIME: 11:50PM

A ten-week-old male infant

CC: Fever

The baby is febrile. His axillary temperature is 101.0°F (38.3°C).

He has no other problem.

Disposition: The mother is advised to give the baby 40mg of Infants' Tylenol and to take him to the ED to be examined.

A ten-week-old infant with any amount of fever (≥ 100.4°F [38.0°C]) should be checked.

## CASE #347

WINTER                                                    TIME: 5:51AM

A four-year-old male child

CC: Insomnia

The child has a behavior problem and he is autistic. His mother states that he wakes up and is playing in the middle of the night. This problem is not new and now appears to be getting worse.

Disposition: The mother is advised to make an appointment to see his pediatrician and a child psychologist for an evaluation and therapy if required. She is also advised regarding sleep regulation and to avoid giving him any caffeinated beverages. The child should sleep every night at the same time and not too early. He should also wake up at the same time each morning. He should sleep in his own bed and in a quiet place without any disturbing light or noise. There should be no screen time for the hour leading up to his bedtime. He should do his bedtime rituals like brushing his teeth, taking a bath, or putting on his pajamas, before going to bed. She could read him a story as well before bed. She should offer him a healthy breakfast in the early morning when he wakes up.

## CASE #348

AUTUMN                                                    TIME: 5:16PM

A three-month-old male infant

CC: Cough & rapid respirations

The infant has had a cough for 2-3 days. He had a fever after having been given immunizations last week. The mother states (via the interpreter) that the infant has been having some rapid respirations with perhaps some retraction under the ribs and is vomiting after the feedings.

Disposition: The mother is advised to take the infant to the ED immediately. She may call 911.

## Case #349

A one-year-old male infant

CC: Cold & touching the ears
The infant has had congestion for 2 days. He has no fever. He touches his ears sometimes.
Disposition: The mother is advised to use Normal Saline nose drops (1-2 drops into the nostrils, three or four times per day for 5-7 days), to offer him more fluid (juice, soup, ginger ale) to drink, to use a humidifier in the room and to observe the infant. If the child were to develop a fever or is being cranky, then he may be seen at the ED, otherwise he is to be checked on Monday (weekend call).

## Case #350

Autumn Time: 8:20PM

A three-year-old male toddler

CC: Head injury
The child fell in the park about 20 minutes ago, and now has a big bump on his forehead. He had no loss of consciousness and no vomiting. The mother states the child wants to sleep. He usually sleeps every evening about this time.
Disposition: The mother is advised to use an ice pack wrapped in a towel on the child's forehead for 10-20 minutes every 15 minutes and to observe. If she suspects that there is unexplained drowsiness, then he is to be seen at the ED.
Also, when he sleeps, she is to make sure he can easily wake up, and that he has no vomiting.

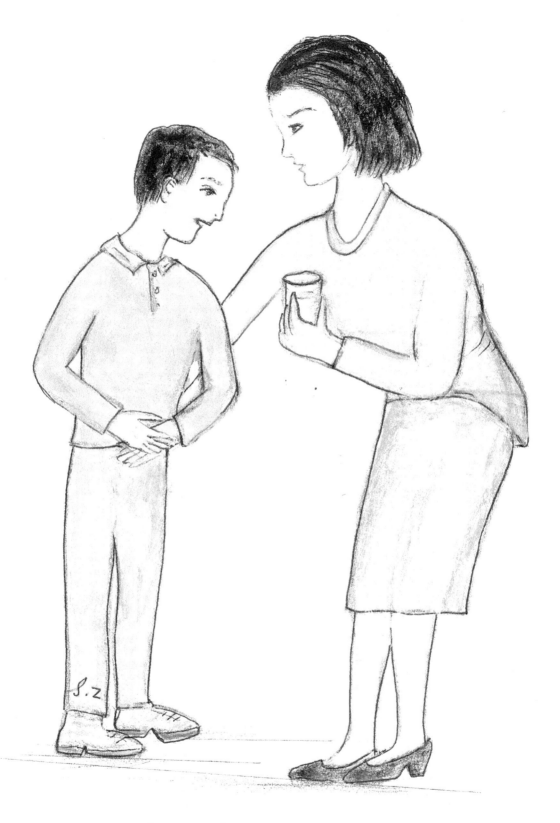

A Child with Abdominal Pain

# Chapter Eight

CASE #351

TIME: 9:00PM

A seven-week-old female infant

CC: Frequent stooling
The infant takes mostly breastmilk and some Enfamil with iron formula as a supplement. She has normal stool according to her mother, but up to 8 times per day. She has only a very small amount of stool each time she defecates; she is otherwise fine.
Disposition: The mother is reassured. Breastfed infants sometimes have several times bowel movements but the stools have normal consistencies and should not be a large amount or very watery. The consistency of stooling is more important than the frequency of stooling in breastfed infants. The stools typically have a yellow-seedy, mustardy semi-solid consistency.

CASE #352

LATE AUTUMN TIME: 8:11AM

A six-year-old male child

CC: Fever & an earache
The child has a fever; his temperature is 101.0ºF (38.3ºC) and he complains of an earache.
Disposition: The mother is advised to give him Children's Tylenol (160mg per 5 mL, 2 teaspoons every 4-6 hours for fever and pain), to offer him fluid (juice, soup, water),

and to call the clinic and take him in to be checked today. The child with fever and an earache has signs of otitis media.

The drug of choice for the treatment of acute otitis media is Amoxicillin 80-90mg/kg per day in divided doses. Children who are allergic to penicillin can be treated with Zithromax 10mg/kg for the first day, then 5mg/kg per day for 4 more days. Omnicef is also an acceptable choice for use in children with otitis media and known penicillin allergy.

## Case #353

Late autumn                                                    Time: 10:55AM

A six-year-old male child

CC: Fever & skin lesions

The child has a fever and lesions over his face and different parts of his legs and neck. His mother states that the child woke up with a large itchy bump on his forehead, and that there are some other bumps that look like mosquito bites on his legs and neck. There is a subjective low-grade fever.

Disposition: The mother is advised regarding giving Children's Tylenol (160mg per 5mL, 2 teaspoons every 4-6 hours) for fever if present and using Calamine lotion for the rash. She may then observe. The child is to be checked if the skin lesions appear in unexposed areas as well, as there is the possibility of his having the chickenpox. If suspecting chickenpox, he should be kept at home and he is not to attend school until all the lesions are scabbed over and dried up. If thought to be insect bites, then the mother is to make sure that the areas surrounding the bites are not very red or hard and painful, as these may be signs of bacterial skin infection. If a secondary skin infection is suspected, then, the child should be checked and receive appropriate antibiotics.

## Case #354

Late autumn                                                    Time: 3:50PM

A seven-year-old male child

CC: Itchy rash

The child has had an itchy rash over his face and hands since yesterday. He has no fever. The mother cannot think of any new exposures.

Disposition: The mother is advised to give him Benadryl liquid (Diphenhydramine HCL12.5mg per 5 mL) one teaspoon every 6-8 hours for the itching, for 3-5 days, to avoid hyper-allergenic foods (eggs, chocolate, strawberry, tomato sauce, seafood/shellfish, peanut butter or peanuts/nuts), and to observe. He is to be checked if the condition persists.

## Case #355

A four-year-old male child

CC: Cough & fever after flu immunization
The child is a known asthmatic and he had his booster immunizations and flu vaccine yesterday. He has a temperature of 102.5°F (39.1°C) today. He has received Children's Motrin (100mg per 5 mL, one and a half teaspoons) for the fever and his temperature is down but he has been having a cough.
Disposition: The mother is advised to start his asthma medicine (albuterol) for his cough, and to offer him more fluid (water, juice, soup, ginger ale) to drink. She could also give him Children's Tylenol (160mg per 5 mL, 6mL every 4-6 hours) for continued fever, and is to observe her son. The influenza vaccine used for asthmatic children is derived from an inactivated virus, tri-valent or quadri-valent, and sometimes the child may develop a fever after receiving the vaccine. Antipyretics and hydration help the child feel better.

## Case #356

A four-year-old male child

CC: Medication refill request
The child is an asthmatic and needs a refill of his albuterol solution for inhalation to use via nebulizer.
Disposition: The medication is ordered by phone to the pharmacy and the mother is advised to pick up the medicine and to use as instructed. I recommended that the mother keep the scheduled appointment for the child's asthma follow-up.

## Case #357

A 23-month-old female toddler

CC: Accidental ingestion (non-food)

The mother states that the child had a bite of the deodorant stick about 20 minutes ago. She has rinsed out the child's mouth and she looks fine now.

Disposition: The mother is advised to call the poison control center at 1-800-222-1222 and to read the content of the deodorant to these experts and receive advice accordingly. She may call us back if needed.

## CASE #358

AUTUMN                                                             TIME: 10:43PM

A two-year-old male toddler

CC: The child has wheezing and breathing problems

The mother was called immediately via the answering service but there was no response. It appears that the child was taken to the ED.

The asthmatic child should always have asthma medicine (albuterol) at home and with the first sign of asthma, like cough and wheezing, the medication is to be started. If the child continues to be symptomatic (coughing, wheezing), then the medication is to be repeated in 20 minutes x 2, and if the child continues to have problem then he or she is to be checked as soon as possible or immediately if in any distress.

## CASE #359

AUTUMN                                                             TIME: 11:14PM

A two-year-old male toddler

CC: wheezing

The child has a cough and wheezing and rapid breathing. He is happy and playful. He had one episode of wheezing previously when he was an infant. His older brother is an asthmatic. There is no asthma medicine available for him. He is in no distress (no retractions, no nasal flaring, and no abdominal breathing).

Disposition: The mother is advised to take him to the hospital as soon as possible. If she feels that he is in distress, she may call 911.

The child currently has rapid breathing and a history of having wheezed and so it is better that he be checked at the ED.

# Case #360

Autumn                                        Time: 7:15AM

A four-year-old male child

CC: Fever & an earache
The child has been having a fever and an earache for 3 days.
Tylenol has been given, but he continues to have both a fever and an earache.
Disposition: The mother is advised to take the child to be checked and receive proper antibiotics. The antibiotic of choice for acute otitis media is Amoxicillin 80-90 mg per kg of body weight per day, divided in 2-3 doses for10 days.

# Case #361

Autumn                                        Time: 8:40AM

A three-year-old female child

CC: Diarrhea & vomiting
The child has diarrhea and vomiting. She has no fever. There is no blood and no mucus in her stool, and there is neither blood nor bile in the vomitus.
Disposition: The mother is advised to offer her Pedialyte in small amounts. She also can offer her some other clear fluids like ginger ale, white grape juice and Gatorade. When she is no longer vomiting, she can be given solid foods (well-cooked white rice, applesauce, banana, plain yogurt) and the child is to be observed. If the child continues with these problems, then she is to be checked. Also, she can be checked if she develops severe episodic abdominal pains, blood in stool, or if she is not voiding at least 3 times a day. Rotavirus infections occur mostly in cooler seasons and day care attendees.

# Case #362

Autumn                                        Time: 10:45AM

A one-month-old female neonate

CC: Excessive crying
The baby had been crying excessively.
The mother was called immediately via the answering service but there was no response.
The neonate with excessive crying that is not consolable should be checked immediately.

## CASE #363

AUTUMN                                                    TIME: 11:40AM

A one-month-old female neonate

CC: Excessive crying & rash and spitting up
The infant has been crying excessively; she also has been having a rash on her body and diaper area for 4 days. Her bowel movement is normal with normal stool color. She is taking formula less than she usually does and is spitting up. She sometimes spits up because of the crying.
Disposition: The father is advised to take the baby to the ED to be checked. The neonate with excessive crying that is not consolable should be checked immediately.

## CASE #364

AUTUMN                                                    TIME: 11:56AM

A two-year-old female toddler

CC: Poor appetite & occasional vomiting
The child does not want to eat, but she has been drinking just juice for the past 2 days. She has had no fever, but she occasionally vomits. There is no blood nor bile in the vomit. She has been having normal bowel movements and is urinating well.
Disposition: The mother is advised to give her Pedialyte and other clear fluids like Gatorade and broth. If she can tolerate these well, then the mother is to offer her soft foods (applesauce, pudding and Jell-O) and to continue the Pedialyte and observe.
She may then gradually introduce regular foods in her diet, and she may also give her Multivitamin drops (Poly-Vi-Sol) one mL daily.
A child taking in only juice for 2 days might become hyponatremic (low blood sodium) and so needs fluids which contain electrolytes like Pedialyte and Gatorade.
The mother may have the toddler examined at the clinic tomorrow (weekend call) if she is urinating well. She may be seen sooner if she is not voiding well, at least three times a day.

## CASE #365

AUTUMN                                                    TIME: 11:57AM

A 13-month-old female toddler

CC: Cough & fever
The child has been coughing a great deal since yesterday afternoon. Also, she had a fever and her temperature was 103.0°F (39.4°C) Tylenol and Motrin were given. She has an underlying history of asthma and albuterol inhalation solution is being used via a nebulizer, but despite this, she continues to cough a great deal.
Disposition: The mother is advised that the albuterol treatment may be repeated in 20 minutes and then every four hours. Also, if the fever is not coming down with the antipyretics and she continues to cough a great deal, then the mother can have her checked at the ED today. Influenza, parainfluenza, respiratory syncytial virus are viruses that are most active in the autumn and cold seasons. When a child is an asthmatic, viral respiratory infections often trigger the asthma.


## CASE #366

AUTUMN                                                    TIME: 12:50PM

A one-month-old female neonate

CC: Stuffy nose
The infant has a stuffy nose and no fever. She is otherwise fine.
Disposition: The mother is advised (via Spanish speaking interpreter) to use Normal Saline nose drops (1-2 drops into the nostrils, three or four times per day for 3-5 days). Also, she is to use a humidifier in the room and to observe the infant. She may call us back if the baby is not improving or if there is a fever (rectal temperature ≥100.4°F[38.0°C]).


## CASE #367

AUTUMN                                                    TIME: 2:46PM

A three-month-old male infant

CC: Vomiting
The infant vomited twice yesterday and once today.
He is taking predominantly breastmilk and then an extra 3 ounces of formula every 2-3 hours. He has been having normal bowel movements and he has no fever. There is neither blood nor bile in the vomitus.
Disposition: His father is advised regarding the feedings. It appears that the baby is

being overfed. The stomach has a capacity of only about 4-5 ounces at this age; and it takes about 3-4 hours for the stomach to empty. Feeding occurring sooner than every 3-4 hours at this age will go atop of the previous one, causing vomiting. The father is advised to give Pedialyte for 2-3 feedings and to observe. He may then have the baby just breastfeed every 3-4 hours. If it appears that the baby is not satiated with breastfeeding alone, then 1-2 oz. of formula can be offered as a supplement. Alternatively, the mother may follow up with a lactation consultant to determine if the formula is even necessary. His father may have the baby checked if his vomiting persists.

## Case #368

AUTUMN                                                          TIME: 4:30PM

A 17-month-old female toddler

CC: Cold & cough
The child has a cold and cough for 4 days. She has been coughing worse at night; she has not had any fever. She has a history of one episode of bronchiolitis in the past and albuterol metered-dose-inhaler (MDI) via spacer had been used. The mother thinks that the child does not need any albuterol now.
Disposition: The mother is advised to give her fluids like juice, soup, and ginger ale. For the cough, she can try the albuterol MDI via the spacer 2 puffs every 4-6 hours, and observe. The mother should continue using the albuterol until she has no cough. A humidifier and Normal Saline nasal spray can also be used. The child may be checked if worsening or not improving or if she were to develop a fever ≥102.2°F (39.0°C).

## Case #369

AUTUMN                                                          TIME: 4:40PM

A four-year-old male child

CC: Fever off-and-on for one week
The child has been having a fever off-and-on since last week. He was seen by his physician five days ago, and mother had been told that he has a viral condition. However, the child continues to have a fever at night.
Disposition: The mother is advised that if the fever persists, then he should be rechecked tomorrow. A fever that is prolonged beyond 5 days and definitely beyond a week requires a more in-depth evaluation. If no source can be identified and it has been persistent over 7 days, then it is a fever of unknown origin (FUO). Among the

causes are infections, autoimmune and oncologic conditions. The most common cause is a hidden infection like sinusitis. A much less common hidden infection may be an abscess formation, like a brain abscess.

## Case #370

AUTUMN                                                        TIME: 6:07PM

A one-year-old female infant

CC: Does not like cow's milk
The mother states that the child does not like milk but she eats food and dairy products. She is otherwise fine.
Disposition: The mother is advised to make sure the infant eats well and drinks enough fluids; she may add flavor to the milk and try or if she prefers, and if the child is growing well, she may just continue to give other full-fat dairy products like yogurts and cheeses, at least 2-3 servings a day. Orange juice with added calcium can also be given, 4-6 oz. daily.

## Case #371

AUTUMN                                                       TIME: 6:36 PM

A five-year-old male child

CC: Nail injury
The child had a finger nail injury few weeks ago. The nail of his right index finger was injured; the nail is separated and is hanging on by the corner.
Disposition: The mother is advised to take care of the nail, by careful removal and to clean the nail bed.

## Case #372

AUTUMN                                                        TIME: 7:34PM

A five-year-old male child

CC: Fever & leg pain
The child has a slight fever and leg pain that started this afternoon.
He has no vomiting, and no other problem. There is no limp.
Disposition: The mother is advised to give him Children's Tylenol (160mg per 5mL,

6mL every4-6 hours) for fever and to observe. The mother may have the child examined tomorrow if the condition persists.

## Case #373

An 18-month-old female toddler

CC: Fever & rash
The child has a slight fever and a rash, both starting today. She looks fine; she has neither vomiting nor any other problem.
She has no known allergies.
Disposition: The father is advised to give her Infants' Tylenol 120mg every 4-6 hours for fever and to use Calamine lotion on the rash if it is itchy and to observe. The father may have the child checked tomorrow.

## Case #374

A two-year-old male toddler

CC: Constipation
The child is constipated. He has neither vomiting nor any other problem.
Disposition: The mother is advised regarding constipation. She may offer the toddler a tablespoon of mineral oil mixed with juice, as well as juices like prune, apricot, pear or peach. Two ounces of these juices may be diluted with 1-2oz. of water, and foods like oatmeal cereal may be given and the child can be observed. Milk and other dairy products should be limited now as they are constipating. Bananas are also constipating, and so other fruits should be given. Mother can follow-up with the pediatrician if these dietary changes do not help the toddler.

## Case #375

A 16-month-old male toddler

CC: Fever
The child has a fever that started today. His temperature was between 101.0-102.0°F

(38.3-38.8°C), Tylenol was given. He has no vomiting nor any other problem. Two weeks prior he had a fever. Then, he was seen by physician and had been told he had a viral infection.

Disposition: The mother is advised to take the child to be checked tomorrow if the fever persists.

## Case #376

Autumn                                                                 Time: 6:50AM

A seven-week-old male infant

CC: Cough
The infant has been coughing for 3 days. He has not had any fever. His bowel movements are normal and he has had no vomiting.

Disposition: The mother is advised to have the baby checked today. A neonate with a cough should be examined.

## Case #377

Autumn                                                                 Time: 6:55AM

A three-year-old female child

CC: Cough & history of asthma
The child has a cough and temperature of 100.0°F (37.7°C).
She has a history of bronchial asthma. She is otherwise fine.

Disposition: The mother is advised to start using her asthma medicine, an albuterol MDI via spacer. Two puffs should be given every 4 hours in the beginning and then when the cough is better, every 6 hours. They should continue using the albuterol until she has no cough at all, even when she is running and with exertion. The mother should offer her more fluids (juice, soup, ginger ale) and give her Children's Tylenol (160mg per 5mL, one teaspoon every 4-6 hours) for fever (for a temperature ≥100.4F [38.0C]), and the child is to be observed.

## Case #378

Winter                                                                 Time: 5:15PM

An eight-month-old female infant

CC: Loose bowel movement & teething

The infant has had loose bowel movements for one or two days and she is also teething. Her mother has been giving her Pedialyte.

Disposition: The mother is advised regarding teething symptoms which could be associated with slight fever and crankiness and loose bowel movements. She can offer her fluids like Pedialyte, white grape juice and foods like rice cereal, applesauce, banana and plain yogurt. She should also continue the breastmilk or formula, and observe.

## CASE #379

WINTER                                          TIME: 5:57PM

A ten-day-old female neonate

CC: Constipation & straining

The baby is constipated, is straining and has a bowel movement only every other day.

Disposition: The mother is advised to offer the neonate boiled then cooled water and to observe. If the baby is comfortable, and the stools are not hard, then not having bowel movement every day is acceptable. The consistency and not the frequency of bowel movements are important. Straining is common in young infants since intra-abdominal pressure and the relaxation of the pelvic floor muscles are not well-coordinated. Also, as they are often in a horizontal position, they do not have the benefit of gravity to assist them with their bowel movement.

## CASE #380

WINTER                                          TIME: 6:17PM

A nine-month-old female infant

CC: Cough

The infant has a cough; she was just seen by a physician and was given Amoxicillin and albuterol syrup. The albuterol syrup is being given at 0.8mL every 8 hours for the cough. His father has a question about the duration of which to use the medications.

Disposition: The father is told that the course of treatment with Amoxicillin for the ear infection is usually 10 days. The albuterol has been given for the cough, and is to be continued if the child is coughing, usually for about 7-10 days.

## Case #381

Winter                                                    Time: 6:35PM

A 12-month-old male infant

CC: The infant has some sores in the mouth, blisters on his lips and red circles on his tongue. He is on Amoxicillin.

Disposition: The mother is advised to offer him soft and mild foods to prevent irritation. She may give him multivitamin drops (Poly-Vi-Sol) 1.0mL daily. If there is a fever, she may give him Infants' Tylenol 80mg every 4-6 hours. She may use this for the mouth pain as well. The mother is also advised to offer the infant some water to drink after each feeding to wash his mouth. Oral Benadryl elixir and oral Maalox can also be used to coat the mouth lesions, so that they do not hurt that much. Enteroviruses like some strains of Coxsackievirus and Echovirus infections can cause mouth lesions and stomatitis in infants and children. If there is concern for Herpes virus infection, then the child can be evaluated by a physician in the morning as long as he is well-hydrated this evening.

## Case #382

Winter                                                    Time: 6:50PM

A six-month-old male infant

CC: Cold symptoms & a fever

The infant has cold symptoms and a fever. His temperature is 101.6°F (38.6°C); Infants' Tylenol 80mg has been given.

Disposition: The mother is advised to use Normal Saline nose drops (1-2 drops into the nostrils three or four times per day for 3-5 days) for the congestion. To help the fever, she may continue to give him Infants' Tylenol 80mg every 4-6 hours (for a temperature ≥100.4°F [38.0°C]), offer more fluid (juice, formula or breast milk), and observe.

## Case #383

Winter                                                    Time: 1:35AM

A one-year-old female infant

CC: Cold symptoms & a fever

The infant has been having a cold for about one week. She started to have a fever today. She has had some loose bowel movements and a few episodes of vomiting.

Disposition: The mother is advised to give the baby Infants' Tylenol 80mg every 4-6 hours for fever, and to offer her more fluids (juice, soup, flat ginger ale). She is also given dietary counselling regarding how to help with the loose bowel movements (rice cereal, applesauce, banana, plain yogurt) and she is to observe the infant. If the fever persists, she is to take the child in to be checked.

## CASE #384

WINTER                                                    TIME: 2:30AM

A three-year-old female toddler

CC: Cough & asthma

The child has been having a cough for three days and she has a history of asthma. She just started to have a fever; her temperature is 102.0°F (38.8°C). Her mother does not have Tylenol.

Disposition: The mother is advised to give her Children's Motrin (100mg per 5mL, 6 mL every 6-8 hours) or Children's Tylenol (160mg per 5 mL, one teaspoon every 4-6 hours) for fever, to start to use her albuterol (albuterol MDI via spacer, 2 puffs every 4 hours in the beginning, and then every 6 hours) for her cough, to offer her fluids (juice, soup, ginger ale), and to observe.

## CASE #385

WINTER                                                    TIME: 7:00AM

A 14-month-old female infant

CC: Diarrhea & vomiting

The infant has been having diarrhea and vomiting for two days. She had several loose bowel movements up until yesterday; she has not had any bowel movements since yesterday afternoon. She vomited the milk once today.

Disposition: The father is advised to get Pedialyte and to offer it to her in small amounts, while making sure she can retain it. Thereafter, he may continue giving her Pedialyte and clear fluids (water, white grape juice, flat ginger ale), and if she still has loose bowel movements thereafter, the father can offer her foods like white rice, applesauce, banana, plain yogurt, and then observe. He may take her to be examined at the clinic later today if he is having difficulty getting her to drink or if she is not urinating at least once every 6-8 hours.

## Case #386

A one-year-old female infant

CC: Cold & cough
The infant has been having a cold and cough for 4 days. At the beginning of this illness, she had a fever and received Infants' Tylenol and Children's Motrin and the fever has since subsided. However, she continues to have a cough.
Disposition: The mother is advised to give her more fluids (water, juice, soup), to use a humidifier in the room, and to observe. She is to have her checked tomorrow in the clinic if the cold is worsening and not improving.

## Case #387

Winter                                                    Time: 8:40AM

A seven-year-old male child

CC: Chickenpox
The mother states that the child appears to have the chickenpox (this is before the era of immunization against chickenpox). The child is not immunized against varicella zoster virus (VZV). He has a fever and tiny itchy skin lesions with fluid in the bumps on different parts of his body, including his chest, neck, and face.
Disposition: The mother is advised to give him Children's Tylenol (160mg per 5mL, 2 teaspoons every 4-6 hours) for the fever and to use Calamine lotion on the skin lesions a few times per day. She should avoid taking him out in public and keep him at home until all the skin lesions dry up and are scabs. They should especially avoid pregnant women and immunocompromised individuals.

## Case #388

Winter                                                    Time: 9:00AM

An eight-year-old female child

CC: Cough

The child has had a cough since yesterday. She was sent home from school because of the cough and a fever. Tylenol was given and the fever subsided. She has no history of asthma.

Disposition: The mother is advised regarding giving fluids (juice, soup, ginger ale) and cough syrup Robitussin DM (one teaspoon three times per day for 3-5 days), and observe. While cough medicine is generally not used for children 6 years and under, it can be helpful for some older children.

## CASE #389

A 13-year-old female adolescent

CC: Medication refill request
The adolescent has a cold and underlying asthma. She has run out of her albuterol inhaler.

Disposition: The pharmacy is called and the medication albuterol metered-dose-inhaler (MDI) is ordered. It is to be used as such: 2 puffs every 4 to 6 hours for cough and wheezing. It is recommended that the mother keep her asthma follow-up appointment.

## CASE #390

A two-year-old male toddler

CC: Medication refill request
The child has a cold and underlying asthma. His mother states that he has run out of the albuterol solution for inhalation via nebulizer.

Disposition: The pharmacy is called and the medication albuterol solution for inhalation is ordered to be used 0.5mL via Nebulizer with Normal Saline inhalation solution 3mL via nebulizer every 4 to 6 hours for cough and wheezing. Normal Saline nose drops and increasing oral fluids is advised, and the toddler is to be observed. It is recommended that the mother keep the asthma follow-up appointment.

## CASE #391

A seven-year-old female child

CC: Fever & headache
The child has a fever and a headache. She has been having a fever for 2 days. Motrin was given last night. She has been under pediatric allergist care for an allergic condition and she has also been on Augmentin for about 6 weeks according to the mother. Disposition: The mother is advised to use Normal Saline nose drops in her nostrils and use her Nasonex nasal spray (one spray in each nostril once daily), Motrin (100mg per 5mL, 2 teaspoons every 6-8 hours) for fever, and to observe to see whether the fever and headache dissipate with these measures. If headaches or fevers persist, then she is to be examined.

## CASE #392
WINTER                                                    TIME: 10:41AM

A five-year-old female child

CC: Fever & an earache and stomachache
The child has had a fever, an earache and a stomachache for a few days. Her temperature has not been taken. Motrin was given and her earache has been off-and-on for a while. Disposition: The mother is advised to give her Children's Tylenol (160mg per 5mL, 2 teaspoons every 4-6 hours) or Children's Motrin (100mg per 5mL, 2 teaspoons every6-8 hours) for fever. She should observe to see if the condition persists, if so then she may be examined at the ED. If the symptoms are controlled, then she may be seen on Monday morning (weekend call).

## CASE #393
WINTER                                                    TIME: 11:18AM

A two-year-old male toddler

CC: Medication refill request
The child is an asthmatic and is low on his asthma medications.
He is on albuterol premixed 0.083% via nebulizer every 4-6 hours for cough and wheezing and Pulmicort inhalation solution 0.25mg/2mL twice per day as instructed. The medication is ordered via phone to the pharmacy and is to be picked up by the parents. The mother is advised to keep the asthma follow-up appointment.

## Case #394

Time: 11:44AM

A seven-year-old male child

CC: Medication refill request
The child is an asthmatic; he has run out of his medicine and has no refills on file.
Disposition: The mother is advised that an albuterol inhaler will be ordered by phone
to the pharmacy to be picked up and it is to be used 2 puffs every 4 to 6 hours for cough
and wheezing. It is recommended that they make an asthma follow-up appointment.

## Case #395

Winter

Time: 12:00PM

A four-year-old female child

CC: Fever & diarrhea
The child has been having a fever and diarrhea off-and-on for about 2 weeks. There is
neither blood nor mucus in stool. Today she has a temperature of 102.0°F (38.8°C),
and she has a cough and is vomiting after coughing. The child also has a history of
asthma
Disposition: The mother is advised to give her Children's Tylenol (160mg per 5mL,
6mL every 4-6 hours) or Children's Motrin (100mg per 5mL, one and a half teaspoons
every 6-8 hours) for the fever. She should also give her Pedialyte and clear fluids (white
grape juice, ginger ale), and use the asthma medicine (albuterol). If the child looks sick,
then she is to be seen at the ED today. Because of duration of the child's diarrhea and
fever, the child should be checked and some laboratory work-up may be warranted.
However, she is likely just developing a new episode of another viral illness, especially
if she has a period of wellness between now and the initial illness.

## Case #396

Winter

Time: 12:10PM

A one-year-old female infant

CC: Fever & vomiting
The infant has had a fever since yesterday and vomited once today. Her bowel movement
is normal. There is no blood and no bile in the vomitus.

Disposition: The mother is advised to give her Infants'Tylenol 80mg every 4-6 hours for fever, to offer her fluids (Pedialyte, white grape juice, and flat ginger ale), and to observe. She is to be examined if the fever persists, especially if the temperature is ≥102.2°F (39.0°C), if mother is not able to keep her hydrated (she should be urinating every 6-8 hours), or if there is a bad smell to the urine.

## CASE #397

WINTER                                                                    TIME: 1:30PM

A two-year-old female toddler

CC: High fever

The child has been having a high fever since yesterday. She was seen at a walk-in clinic and the mother has been advised about how to control the fever. The toddler has had no diarrhea and no vomiting, but she is refusing to drink fluids. She has not urinated yet today.

Disposition: The mother is advised to give her clear fluids (water, juice, ginger ale) and Children's Motrin (100mg per 5mL, 6 mL for fever every 6-8 hours) and if need be Children'sTylenol (160mg per 5mL, 5mL for fever every 4-6 hours) and to observe. If she is not urinating after being given fluids or if the fever persists despite antipyretics, then she is to take her to the ED.

## CASE #398

WINTER                                                                    TIME: 2:40PM

A six-month-old female infant

CC: Medication question

There was a call from pharmacy regarding a request for clarification of two prescriptions for Amoxicillin 250mg/5mL and Normal Saline nose drops that were given yesterday, the details of each were confirmed.

## CASE #399

WINTER                                                                    TIME 4:16PM

An eight-month-old male infant

CC: Eye congestion & eye discharge

The infant has been congested. His eyes are also congested since yesterday and he is having greenish mucus coming out from his eyes. He has had no fever. He has been having medicine via nebulizer.

Disposition: The mother is advised regarding eye hygiene (she is to clean the eyelids gently with sterile water and cotton balls) and a prescription is given via the pharmacy for him to receive Gentamycin ophthalmic drops to be used 1-2 drops into the eyes, every 6 hours for 5-7 days. She is to observe and see that he is improving but to also to obtain an appointment for follow-up at the clinic tomorrow (weekend call), as this baby's ears should be checked as well, given his young age.

## CASE #400

WINTER                                                              TIME: 7:25PM

A ten-day-old male neonate

CC: Constipation

The baby is constipated. He has not had any bowel movements for two days. He has had no vomiting and his abdomen appears fine. The consistency of his last bowel movement was normal.

Disposition: The mother is advised to offer him cooled previously boiled water, to make sure he is taking enough breastmilk or formula, and to observe. She may also massage his abdomen in a clockwise fashion, bicycle the legs, and gently take a rectal temperature using a little bit of Vaseline with the thermometer. The consistency of the bowel movements is more important than the frequency of the bowel movements at this age.

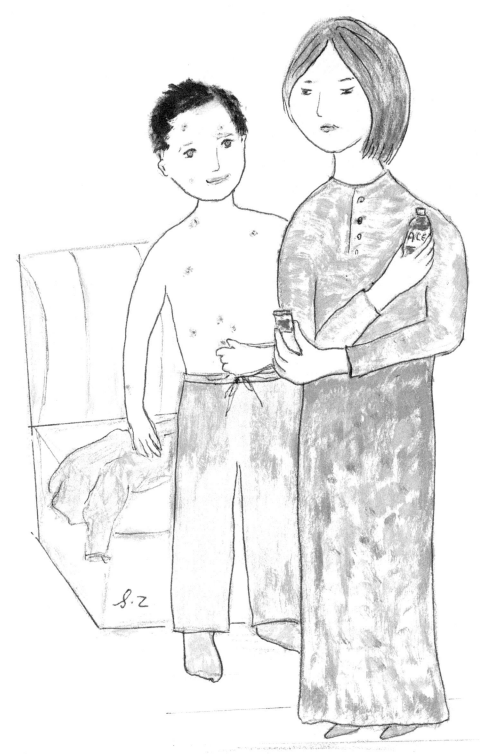

A Child with ChickenPox

# CHAPTER NINE

———◦∾◦———

## CASE #401

TIME: 11:30PM

A two-year-old male toddler

CC: Toxic accidental ingestion

The child ingested one or two tablets of Percocet about 20 minutes ago. According to the mother, she called the poison control center and was advised to call the doctor. The mother had no syrup of ipecac and could not induce vomiting. This syrup used to be recommended (1965-2003) as a method of inducing vomiting in cases of accidental poisoning. However, currently, the American Academy of Pediatrics (AAP) no longer advises, and in fact strongly advises against the use of syrup of ipecac. The AAP further recommends that any syrup of ipecac in the home be disposed of, as there has been no evidence that it helps and some evidence of harm in some cases from its use.

Disposition: The mother is advised to take the child to the ED immediately (she may call 911).

Percocet is a combination of oxycodone and acetaminophen. The possibility of respiratory depression and hypotension from the accidental ingestion of narcotics in a two-year-old child leads to the immediate need to be seen at the ED. Poison Control can be reached at 1-800-222-1222. It is not clear if the mother in fact called this center or if she misunderstood their instructions.

## CASE #402

WINTER  TIME:10: 29PM

A one-year-old male infant

CC: High fever
The infant has a fever; his temperature is 104.0°F (40.0°C). Motrin (ibuprofen) has just been given. The infant has been having a cold for several days and has now developed a fever and he has also vomited one time today.

Disposition: The mother is advised to give him Infants' Tylenol 80mg every 4-6 hours or Children's Motrin (100mg per 5mL, one teaspoon every 6-8 hours) for fever and to offer him clear fluids (water, juice, Pedialyte). However, if the fever persists, then she is to have the baby checked at the ED, given his young age and the height of the fever. As the child had a cold for several days already, there is a possibility of his having developed a secondary bacterial infection, given the timing and height of the fever, and so the child should be checked.

# CASE #403

WINTER                                                          TIME: 10:00PM

A Six-month-old female infant

CC: Bloody diarrhea
The infant has bloody diarrhea. She was recently hospitalized for a urinary tract infection (UTI). There, she had received IV fluids and IV antibiotics and she was just send home today. However, since discharged she has developed bloody diarrhea.

Disposition: The mother is advised to take the infant back to the hospital for an examination and a primary laboratory workup: a stool test for culture, ova and parasite and a complete blood count (CBC) is to be done.

Also, as she has been on antibiotics for a period, the possibility of Clostridium difficile infection in the intestines should also be considered. However, in children under the age of one year this is more difficult to diagnose as often infants are colonized with this bacterium.

# CASE #404

WINTER                                                          TIME: 10:10PM

A 16-year-old female adolescent

CC: Hair loss
The adolescent states that her hair is falling out and that she has bald spots on her scalp.

Disposition: The adolescent girl is advised to be checked during the daytime and on a weekday at the clinic. She may need a laboratory workup including thyroid function tests.

## Case #405

A four-month-old female infant

CC: Nasal congestion

The infant has been having nasal congestion for about one week. She occasionally vomits as well. She has had no fever and no diarrhea. She is taking formula well, about 5 ounces every 3 hours. Her mother has been using Normal Saline nose drops in her nostrils but she has nasal congestion and has been slightly cranky.

Disposition: The mother is advised to use a humidifier in the room and, if the baby has no fever, continues to feed well, and is not too cranky, then the mother is to wait and have her checked on Monday (weekend call).

## Case #406
Winter                                                  Time: 2:30AM

A one-year-old male infant

CC: Cold symptoms & eye discharge

The infant has been having a cold for 3 days with a runny nose, cough, and eye discharge. There is no redness to the eyes and there has been no mattering of the lashes from the discharge. He had a fever today. He last received a dose of Tylenol eight hours ago.

Disposition: The grandmother is advised regarding the use of Infants' Tylenol, 80mg every 4-6 hours for fever. She is to give him fluids (water, juice, soup, flat ginger ale), clean the eyes with sterile water, and to observe the child. If the condition were to persist, then she is to take the child in to be checked. An eye culture may be done and antibiotic eye drops or eye ointment may be prescribed if required. Also, the baby's ears should be checked to rule out concomitant ear infection.

## Case #407
Winter                                                  Time: 7:41AM

A three-year-old male toddler

CC: Fever & leg pain, refusing to walk

The child has been having a fever for the past 5 days. His temperature is 102.9°F (39.3°C) today and the temperature has been up and down. Today he cannot walk and is complaining that his legs hurt. The mother has not noticed any apparent swelling or changes to the legs.

Disposition: The mother is advised to take the child to the ED to be checked today. A complete history and physical exam including checking the child's hips, knees and ankles as well as the muscles and bones and reflexes should be done; a primary laboratory workup to be done as required (a complete blood count, inflammatory markers, and a possible blood culture). A child with a limp, especially when accompanied by a fever, must be checked.

## Case #408

Winter                                                        Time: 6:30PM

A 16-month-old male infant

CC: Cough & a history of asthma

The infant has a history of asthma; he started coughing today. He is in no distress, has no fever, and has been eating well and is active and playful.

Disposition: The mother is advised to start using the asthma medicine (albuterol) as instructed, and to continue to use the medicine every 4-6 hours until he has no cough at all (if the cough is triggered by a virus, then the cough will usually be present for around 10 days). If he is not getting better with the albuterol, she may call us back.

## Case #409

Winter                                                        Time: 6:41PM

A one-year-old female infant

CC: Fever & cough

The infant has had a fever of 103.0°F (39.4°C) and developed a cough in the past few days. The mother had been given advice previously and the infant is getting better. The fever has now resolved. The mother now has a question regarding the diet and wants to know what she can feed her.

Disposition: The mother is advised that the child may have a regular simple diet with more fluids (juice, soup, flat ginger ale) and less milk as she feels it contributes to her having more phlegm.

## Case #410

A four-year-old male child

CC: Diarrhea & vomiting

The child now has diarrhea and vomiting. His mother states the child had a fever and rash on his body last week. He was seen by his physician and received a penicillin injection. He then developed diarrhea and vomiting. There is no blood in neither the vomitus nor the stool. He is voiding well.

Disposition: His mother is advised to give him Pedialyte and clear fluids (white grape juice, flat ginger ale). When he is no longer vomiting, then she may put him on a diet to help alleviate the diarrhea consisting of soft rice and starchy foods to harden the stools, saltine or graham crackers, applesauce, banana and plain yogurt. She is not to give him any milk for a few days, and in 2 days he can have hard-boiled egg (not fried) and well-cooked white meat (chicken, turkey breast). The child most likely has developed a viral condition. The mother should observe and make sure the child is improving. If not, he should be checked.

## Case #411

A one-year-old male infant

CC: Cough & a history of asthma

The infant has a cough and he has history of asthma. He has had a fever and a cough for the past 2-3 days. He was seen at hospital and he is on Amoxicillin, Prelone (prednisolone) and albuterol solution for inhalation to be used via nebulizer. The child no longer has a fever but he still has a cough.

Disposition: The mother is advised to keep using the medicines as instructed; she is to offer him fluids (juice, soup, flat ginger ale) and observe. The mother is informed that by using the asthma medicine (albuterol every 4-6 hours) and Prelone, the cough will gradually dissipate. The mother should keep the follow up appointment.

## Case #412

A 9-month-old female infant

CC: Fever & mild diarrhea

The infant has been having a fever off and on for 3 days. Infants' Tylenol was given to her two times yesterday and once today, about 9 hours ago, but the fever has returned. She also had loose bowel movements yesterday.

Disposition: The mother is advised to take the temperature and give her Infants' Tylenol 80mg every 4-6 hours for fever (temperature ≥100.4°F [38.0°C]) and to offer her more fluids (water, juice, broth) and observe. If the problem persists, the infant is to be checked. A slight fever associated with loose bowel movements could be explained by the eruption of teeth (teething). If the fever is ≥102.2°F (39.0°C), then it is better to have the baby checked.

## Case #413

Winter                                    Time: 11:00PM

A one-year-old female infant

CC: Cough & fever

The infant has been having a cough and a fever. Infants' Tylenol was given 2 hours ago, and currently she has no fever; but she has been coughing. Her parents had flu symptoms recently; the infant has no history of asthma.

Disposition: The father is advised to offer her fluids (warm soup, juice, flat ginger ale) and to use Normal Saline nose drops 1-2 drops into the nostrils 3-4 times per day, also to use a humidifier around her, and to observe. He may have her checked tomorrow if required.

## Case #414

Winter                                    Time: 6:38AM

A one-year-old male infant

CC: High fever & cough and heavy mucus from the nose

The infant has a fever; his temperature is 104.0°F (40.0°C) this morning. He had a fever 5 days ago; he was seen at the ED then and diagnosed as having a viral infection.

The use of Motrin and Tylenol was advised. Since then, the child has been coughing and he now has heavy mucus from his nose.

Disposition: The mother is advised to give him Children's Motrin (100mg per 5mL, one teaspoon every 6-8 hours) for fever and to offer him fluids (juice, soup, flat ginger ale). She is to take him to be reexamined today. The infant should be checked because of the high fever and heavy mucus. There is the possibility of his having a secondary bacterial infection and that he may require antibiotics.

## CASE #415

LATE SPRING                                          TIME: 5:37PM

A two-year-old male toddler

CC: Eye discharge

The child has eye discharge today. He has been having a cold for 5 days. He has no fever.

Disposition: The father is advised regarding eye hygiene (clean the eyes with sterile water) and is advised to have the toddler checked tomorrow. The child's eyes and ears to be checked as well as the rest of his body.

## CASE #416

LATE SPRING                                          TIME: 5:40PM

A six-month-old female infant

CC: Cough & phlegm

The infant has been having a cough, phlegm, and a problem with bowel movements. She was seen by a physician yesterday.

Disposition: The mother is advised regarding diet and fluids (water, juice and formula or breast milk) and advised to use Normal Saline nose drops 1-2 drops into the nostrils 3-4 times per day for 3-5 days, a humidifier around the baby, and to observe. If the cold is not getting better or if she were to have a temperature ≥102.2°F (39.0°C), she may be reexamined.

## CASE #417

LATE SPRING                                          TIME: 6:08PM

A four-week-old male neonate

CC: Cough & spitting up

The neonate has been coughing, he spits up and his mother noticed blood on the nipple; he also has diarrhea.

Disposition: The mother is advised to take him to the ED to be examined. A neonate with a cough, spitting up and possible bloody vomitus should be checked early.

## Case #418
Late spring                                                  Time: 6:28PM

A three-year-old male toddler

CC: High fever & high white blood cell count

The child has a high fever. He has been sick for the last four days; he was seen by a physician two times since his fever started. His temperature is 104.6°F (40.3°C) today. His mother states that she was told that the white cells in his blood count were high. He is not on any antibiotics.

Disposition: The mother is advised to give him Children's Motrin (100mg per 5mL, 6mL every 6-8 hours) for fever, fluids (water, juice, soup, flat ginger ale), and to have him reexamined tonight if the fever persists.

An elevated white blood cell count is usually a sign of a bacterial infection and a differential test of the white counts should be checked. If there is a shift to the left and the neutrophils or polymorphonuclears (PMNs) are high, that may imply that a bacterial infection is present and treatment with an antibiotic may be necessary.

## Case #419
Late spring                                                  Time: 6:35PM

A two-year-old male toddler

CC: Chickenpox

The child has skin lesions that look like pimples on his chin. He had a fever yesterday. He also has a tiny lesion on his leg. He was exposed to the chickenpox last month.

Disposition: The mother is advised regarding the use of Children's Tylenol (160mg/5mL, one teaspoon every 4-6 hours) for fever and Calamine lotion (for external use) for the itch. The toddler is to be examined tomorrow if required.

The incubation period of varicella infection (chickenpox) is usually 14-16 days, but is occasionally prolonged to 28 days. In temperate climates, the highest prevalence of varicella virus infection is in late winter and early springtime.

# Case #420

Late spring                                          Time: 7:15PM

An eight-month-old female infant

CC: Frequent stooling
The infant has been having diarrhea for two or three days. She has had no vomiting
nor any fever. Her bowel movements are loose, and in small amounts. However, the
frequency of defecation is about seven or eight times per day.
Disposition: The mother is advised to offer the infant some Pedialyte and clear fluids.
She is to also offer her foods like rice cereal, applesauce, banana and plain yogurt and is
to observe. She may be examined tomorrow if required. Some breastfed infants might
have several bowel movements daily, but these should not be voluminous and watery.
Also, at the time of teething, infants might have loose bowel movements and more
frequent stools than usual.

# Case #421

Late spring                                          Time: 10:23PM

A seven-month-old male infant

CC: Cold symptoms & eye discharge
The infant has had cold symptoms for two days. He has a fever; today his temperature
is 100.9°F (38.2°C). He also has some eye discharge. He has neither vomiting nor
diarrhea.
Disposition: The mother is advised regarding Infants' Tylenol 80mg every 4-6 hours
for fever (temperature ≥100.4°F [38.0°C]) and she is to offer him more fluid like
water, juice, formula or breastmilk. Likewise, the mother is advised to clean the eyes
gently with a cotton ball and sterile water and to have the infant checked tomorrow.
Some adenoviral infections are associated with cold symptoms and conjunctivitis.

# Case #422

Late spring                                          Time: 11:30PM

A six-month-old female infant

CC: Question about the dose of Amoxicillin
The infant was checked in the ED today and she is on Amoxicillin for the treatment of

an ear infection. The mother wanted to confirm the dose of the medication.
Disposition: The mother is advised that the dose of Amoxicillin depends on the type and severity of the infection. In children, Amoxicillin may be given at a dose of 45-90 mg/kg body weight per day, and is divided into two or three doses per day. For the treatment of acute otitis media, the higher dose (80-90mg/kg body weight per day) is recommended. The mother is advised to keep the appointment for follow-up of the ear infection.

## CASE #423

LATE SPRING                                                      TIME: 11:38PM

A four-year-old female child

CC: Fever, sore throat, & a stomachache
The child started to have a fever tonight. She has been complaining of a sore throat and stomachache. She has had no vomiting. Her mother has given her Tylenol and she is presently sleeping.
Disposition: The mother is advised to give her Children's Tylenol (160mg/5mL, 6mL every 4-6 hours) for fever and to offer her fluids (juice, soup, ginger ale). She is to have her checked tomorrow morning. The child should be checked for Strep throat.

## CASE #424

LATE SPRING                                                       TIME: 6:40AM

A ten-month-old female infant

CC: Cough
The infant has a cough. She has been coughing a great deal. She was seen at the ED and received an asthma treatment. She was sent home with Motrin only.
Disposition: The mother is advised to offer her fluids (water, juice and formula or breastmilk) and Children's Motrin (100mg/5mL, 3 mL every 6-8 hours) for fever and to use Normal Saline nose drops 1-2 drops into her nostrils, 3-4 times per day. She is also advised to use a humidifier around her and to observe. If the infant has wheezing or was told that she has asthma, then the mother should have the infant rechecked to see if she needs asthma medicine for use at home.

## CASE #425

SUMMER                                                            TIME: 4:50PM

A one-month-old female neonate

CC: Facial rash

The mother states that the baby has a facial rash. She was seen by a physician and received Hydrocortisone ointment, but despite using the Hydrocortisone ointment the problem has persisted. The child was reexamined, the formula was changed to soy formula, and she has been given two feedings, but the problem persists.

Disposition: The mother is advised not to use soap on the baby's face, to continue the soy milk for a few days more (for at least 1-2 weeks) and to observe. If the facial rash is not improving, the mother can try a protein hydrolysate formula like Nutramigen and observe. She may be rechecked sooner if she feels that the rash is worsening.

## CASE #426
SUMMER                                                                TIME: 5:43PM

A seven-month-old male infant

CC: Diarrhea

The infant started to have diarrhea today. On two occasions, he had very loose and large amounts of stool. He has been on antibiotics for about one week. There is neither blood nor mucus in the stool; he has no fever and no vomiting.

Disposition: The mother is advised to give him Pedialyte instead of the formula for a few feedings, and then when he is getting better she is to to give him Lactose-free formula, rice cereal, applesauce and plain yogurt and observe. The mother also is advised to stop the antibiotics and have the infant checked tomorrow.

## CASE #427
SUMMER                                                                TIME: 6:14PM

An eight-week-old female infant

CC: Stuffy nose

The infant has a stuffy nose. She was born prematurely. She was seen at the ED yesterday and was told that she was okay.

Disposition: The mother is advised to use Normal Saline nose drops (1-2 drops into the nostrils three or four times per day for 3-5 days), to use a humidifier around her, and to observe.

SUMMER                                                          TIME: 7:52PM

A ten-month-old female infant

CC: Nasal congestion
The infant has nasal congestion and noisy breathing. She has no family history of asthma and has neither cough nor vomiting.
Disposition: The father is advised to give her more fluid (water, juice, and formula or breastmilk) and to use Normal Saline nose drops in her nostrils (1-2 drops, 3-4 times/day for 3-5 days), to use a humidifier in the room, and to observe.

CASE #429

SUMMER                                                          TIME: 8:22PM

A three-month-old female infant

CC: Constipation
The infant is constipated. She has not moved her bowels today. She has neither vomiting nor any other problems.
Disposition: The mother is advised via a Spanish speaking interpreter to offer her water and small amounts of juices like prune, apricot or pear juice, diluted with water (one ounce of juice and 2-3 oz. water) and to observe.

CASE #430

SUMMER                                                          TIME: 11:57PM

A three-month-old male infant

CC: Cough
The infant has congestion, coughs a great deal, and is vomiting. He has no fever. His temperature has not been taken.
Disposition: His mother is advised that if the child is coughing a great deal or has wheezing (noisy breathing from his chest), then he should be checked at the ED tonight.
The 3-month-old infant with a great deal of coughing should be checked early.
Respiratory syncytial virus (RSV) infection usually occurs during the winter and early spring time. During the summer time, there is the possibility of having bronchiolitis

with other viruses such as Enteroviruses (mostly between June and October) and Adenoviruses (throughout the year). Also, the possibility of aspiration pneumonia and bacterial infections (such as Bordetella Pertussis, Chlamydia Trachomatis and Mycoplasma Pneumoniae [less common at this age]) should be considered.

## CASE #431

SUMMER                                              TIME: 9:18PM

An eight-year-old male child

CC: Cerebral Palsy & possible fever

The child has cerebral palsy. He has been having a fever today. Motrin was given in the morning and Tylenol was given in the afternoon. He has vomited the Tylenol. His rectal temperature is 99.6°F; he refuses to drink Pedialyte.

Disposition: The mother is advised regarding fever. Temperatures between 96.8°F (36°C) up to 100.3°F (37.9°C) that are taken via the mouth or rectum are normal temperatures, and so are not considered to be a fever. Also, she can offer him other fluids (white grape juice, Gatorade), and observe him. The child is to be checked if required (if having a true fever, if refusing to drink anything, or if the mother is concerned).

## CASE #432

SUMMER                                              TIME: 9:48PM

A three-year-old male toddler

CC: Fever

The child had a fever last night. Motrin was given and the fever subsided, but he has developed a rash today. He has no fever but he complained of a sore throat; he has no vomiting.

Disposition: The mother is advised to make sure the child drinks well and to observe. The mother also is advised to have him checked on Monday if required (weekend call). Infections with Enterovirus occur mostly in the summertime and some are associated with fever and non-specific exanthemas.

## CASE #433

SUMMER                                              TIME: 8:30AM

A two-year-old female toddler

CC: Eye congestion

The child has been having eye congestion for about two weeks. The mother denies any eye discharge, no mucus; she has no fever and no other problem.

Disposition: The mother is advised regarding eye hygiene to wash the eyes with cool sterile water and to have the child checked.

Kawasaki disease is associated with bilateral bulbar conjunctival congestion without exudate; but the patient with Kawasaki disease has a fever. In Kawasaki disease, the fever lasts more than 5 days, and there are other symptoms like red and cracked lips, scarlatiniform rash, and cervical lymphadenopathy that are seen in the most cases.

Eye congestion without any other symptoms could be because of irritation by chlorinated water (swimming pool water) or sun exposure.

## CASE #434

SUMMER                                                        TIME: 10:15AM

A seven-month-old female infant

CC: Constipation

The infant is constipated. She has not had any bowel movements for two or three days. She has no vomiting and she is not cranky.

Disposition: The mother is advised to offer her more fluids (water, prune juice, or pear juice). The mother may dilute the juice with water (she may combine 1-2 oz. of juice and 2-3oz. of water) and she is to offer her oatmeal cereal instead of rice cereal and observe the infant.

## CASE #435

SUMMER                                                        TIME: 1:15PM

A two-year-old female toddler

CC: Diarrhea

The child has been having loose stools for about two weeks and no other problems. The mother denies any mucus in stool and there is no visible blood in the stool.

Disposition: The mother is advised regarding the diet. She may stop giving her cow's milk for a few days and instead offer her clear fluid (Pedialyte, white grape juice, Gatorade), and starchy foods like rice, pasta, mashed potato (without butter). She may also offer her applesauce, banana, plain yogurt and observe the toddler. If the stool is a large amount, too watery, or if there is any blood or mucus in the stool, then she may have the toddler checked.

## CASE #436

SUMMER                                                    TIME: 5:01PM

A seven-year-old female child

CC: Needs a dental check-up
The child needs dental work and prophylaxis for prevention of dental cavities.
Disposition: The mother is advised to make an appointment with the dentist to receive dental care.
Children should have regular dental check-ups and fluoride application with fluoride varnish by the dentist. They should have good oral hygiene and avoid sugary drinks and too much sweet foods to prevent dental cavities. Now, some pediatricians' offices offer fluoride varnish application at the 9 month and 18-month well-child visits.

## CASE #437

SUMMER                                                    TIME: 5:10PM

A two-week-old male neonate

CC: Constipation & excessive crying
The neonate had no bowel movements for two days and now has excessive crying.
Disposition: The mother is advised to take the neonate to the ED.
The neonate with constipation and excessive crying should be checked.

## CASE #438

SUMMER                                                    TIME: 9:40PM

A three-week-old female neonate

CC: Feeding question
The father states that the baby wants to be fed every half an hour or every hour.
Disposition: The father is advised regarding newborn feedings. In the beginning, the newborn baby can be fed on demand but soon after, the feedings may be scheduled. This neonate is on formula and may have 2-3 ounces of formula every 2-3 hours and the

caregiver to make sure the nipple of the bottle is appropriate and that the baby is able to suckle the formula well. Then, the parents may gradually increase the amount of formula in each feeding and extend the time between two feedings. The father is also advised to keep the follow-up appointment to make sure the baby is gaining weight properly.

## CASE #439
SUMMER                                                          TIME: 9:30PM

An 11-month-old male infant

CC: Fever
The infant has a fever. His temperature is currently 103.7°F (39.8°C). He was seen by a physician yesterday and his parents were told that he has bilateral otitis media (both ears are infected) and an antibiotic (Augmentin) was prescribed but the parents could not obtain it and so it was not started. Motrin was given, but it has not been effective at reducing the temperature.
Disposition: The parents are advised to take the infant to the ED.
An infant with high fever and acute otitis media should receive antibiotics and as they could not obtain it, the child should be seen and receive an antibiotic injection.

## CASE #440
SUMMER                                                          TIME: 3:00AM

A seven-month-old male infant

CC: Slight cough & loud breathing transiently
The infant has been having a slight cough since yesterday. His mother noticed that the baby's breathing was loud for a few second and then he coughed and woke up. Now, he is fine and is not in any distress. He has no fever and no other problems.
Disposition: The mother is advised regarding wheezing and rapid breathing. The baby is to be observed and to be checked if required.
If the baby has flaring of the nasal alae (outer part of each nostrils), retraction of the skin under the ribs or between or above the ribs, then the mother should have him checked in the ED.

## CASE #441
SUMMER                                                          TIME: 5:15AM

A two-week-old male neonate

CC: Constipation & oral thrush
The baby is constipated and had excessive crying yesterday. He was seen at the ED yesterday. Today she has trouble swallowing because of white spots (oral thrush) in his mouth. They have medication for this.
Disposition: The father is advised to use the medication for the treatment of thrush properly on the spots in the baby's mouth four times per day and that the baby should swallow the medicine. He should continue the medicine until the white spots in the mouth clear up completely and continue the medication for 2-3 days more. If the baby is breastfed, then the mother may use the medication onto her breasts as well. For the constipation, the father may offer the baby some cool boiled water to drink and observe.

## CASE #442

SUMMER                                                    TIME: 5:23PM

A five-week-old female infant

CC: Cold symptoms
The baby has been having a cold for two days. Her nose is congested. She is feeding well and voiding normally.
Disposition: The mother is advised to use Normal Saline nose drops 1-2 drops into the nostrils, 3-4 times per day for 3-5 days, and to use a humidifier in the room and to observe.
If the baby were to have a fever, breathing problems, or vomiting then the mother is to have her infant checked.

## CASE #443

AUTUMN                                                    TIME: 7:38AM

A ten-week-old male infant

CC: Fever
The infant had been exclusively breastfed but formula was introduced today. He started to have a slight fever, a temperature 100.4-100.5°F (38.0-38.05°C) today following his having taken formula. He has also been having frequent bowel movements.
Disposition: The mother is advised to take the infant to be checked today. A young

infant with any fever should be checked.

## Case #444

A six-year-old male child

CC: Fever & sore throat

The child has a fever and a sore throat that started last night. His temperature comes down after taking Motrin, but it rises again.

Disposition: The father is advised to offer him fluids (juice, soup, ginger ale) and Children's Motrin (100mg/5mL, 2 teaspoons every 6-8 hours) for fever and to observe. If the fever and sore throat persist, then the father is to take the child to be checked.

## Case #445

A 21-month-old male toddler

CC: Skin tag

The mother states that the child has had a whitish skin tag on his left shoulder that she thinks appears pinkish today. It is not painful.

Disposition: The mother is advised to keep his skin clean and to observe. If it appears red or painful or if there is any fever, then the toddler is to be checked soon. Otherwise, she may wait until Monday (weekend call) to have him seen.

## Case #446

A two-month-old female infant

CC: Question about medication

The infant had her immunizations today. Her mother thinks she has a fever and she has given her a dose of Tylenol as was instructed and she wants to know if she can also give her Motrin. The baby is otherwise well. She has been feeding well. There is no cough. There is no vomiting.

Disposition: The mother is advised that Children's Motrin is not recommended for infants below six months of age. She can give the Infants' Tylenol 40mg every 4-6 hours for fever. A temperature up to 100.4ºF (38.0ºC) is acceptable but if higher than this, she could give the Infants' Tylenol.

## CASE #447

AUTUMN                                                    TIME: 11:18PM

A four-month-old male infant

CC: Diarrhea
The infant has diarrhea that started today; he has neither fever nor vomiting. There is no mucus and no blood in the stool. He has had three or four loose and watery stools. Disposition: The mother is advised to offer the infant Pedialyte for a few feedings and then to offer him Lactose-free formula, and to observe. If the condition persists, he may be checked.

## CASE #448

AUTUMN                                                    TIME: 9:00PM

A three-week-old female neonate

CC: Vomiting of the formula
The baby has vomited the formula one time this evening. She has neither fever nor any breathing problems. She has had a normal bowel movement tonight.
Disposition: The mother is advised to offer the baby Pedialyte and observe. Reflux precautions are discussed. If she continues to vomit or is cranky, then she is to be checked at the ED.

## CASE #449

AUTUMN                                                    TIME: 10:26PM

A three-month-old female infant

CC: Constipation
The infant has been constipated. She has no vomiting. She has not had any bowel movements for two days. Her abdomen is soft.
Disposition: The mother is advised to offer the infant water and small amounts of juices like prune or pear juice. She may dilute the juice with water (one ounce of juice and 2oz. water) and observe. She also can use the rectal thermometer, lubricated with a

little Vaseline, and gently take a rectal temperature to stimulate the infant's rectum. If there is vomiting or excessive crankiness, then the infant is to be checked.

## Case #450

A 17-month-old male toddler

CC: Ear infection

The child has an ear infection. He was checked by his physician and is on an antibiotic, but he has a cough. He has neither wheezing nor history of asthma.

Disposition: The mother is advised that a cough commonly accompanies an ear infection. She should continue giving him the antibiotics as instructed, offer him more fluids (juice, soup, and flat ginger ale), observe him, and keep his appointment for the follow- up of his ear infection. If two or three days pass while on antibiotics and she feels that the child is not improving, then she may seek follow-up at that point.

There are cough receptors in the tympanic membranes (eardrums); and an inflammation of the eardrum causes cough.

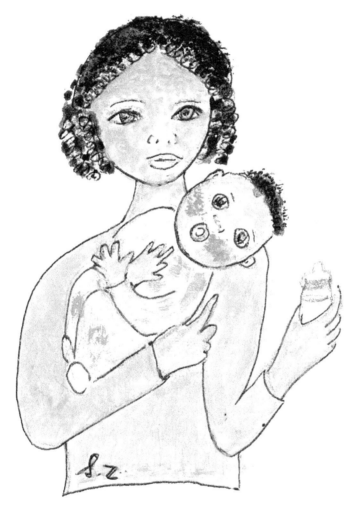

An infant with facial rash

# CHAPTER TEN

~∿~

## CASE #451

AUTUMN                                                    TIME: 11:30PM

An eight-day-old male neonate

CC: Constipation
The baby is constipated. His last bowel movement was yesterday. It was soft, yellow, and seedy in nature. Also, his umbilical cord stump is falling off and it has some bleeding. Disposition: The mother is advised to keep the umbilical area clean with rubbing alcohol and to put a piece of sterile gauze or a bandage on it. The mother is told that the frequency of the bowel movement is less important than the consistency of the bowel movements and that the baby to be observed.
The neonate might not have bowel movements every day, but if the baby is comfortable, has no vomiting, and has a soft abdomen then it is acceptable for the baby not to have a daily bowel movement.

## CASE #452

AUTUMN                                                    TIME: 8:30AM

A special-needs child

CC: The foster mother called to inform the physician's office that the child had a leaking tube and wheezing and has been taken to the hospital. This call was just to pass along this information.
A special-needs child usually has multiple problems and it is acceptable to seek medical

attention as soon as required.

## Case #453

Time: 12:30PM

A one-month-old female neonate

CC: Cold symptoms
The baby has been sneezing and has had a cough for two days. Her temperature has been normal. She has been feeding well and has been voiding normally.
Disposition: The mother is advised that if the baby looks fine, has no fever, no vomiting and is not in any distress, she can use Normal Saline nose drops (1-2 drops into the nostrils, 3-4 times per day for 3-5 days), use a humidifier in the room, and is to observe the baby. The mother may take the baby to be checked tomorrow if required.

## Case #454

Autumn                                                      Time: 1:30PM

A three-month-old female infant

CC: Rash
The infant has a rough, peeling rash on her trunk for the last two to three days. Her mother denies introducing any new foods to the baby's diet and she is breastfed.
Disposition: The mother is advised to avoid consuming hyper-allergenic foods (cow's milk, eggs, chocolate, tomato sauce, seafood) that may affect the breastmilk. She should also refrain from using soap on the baby's body every day, and is to observe the baby. The infant may be checked in the clinic.

## Case #455

Autumn                                                      Time: 3:00PM

A two-month-old female infant

CC: Fever
The infant has been having a fever today. Her temperature was 102.0°F (38.8°C) this morning and she received 80mg of Infants' Tylenol drops. Currently her temperature is 101.0°F (38.3°C). She has been cranky.
Disposition: The mother is advised regarding the appropriate dose of the Infants'

Tylenol (which for a two-month-old infant is 40mg every 4-6 hours) and the mother is advised to take the infant to the ED to be checked today. A 2-month-old infant with a fever should be checked as soon as possible.

## Case #456

Autumn                                                    Time: 8:00PM

A six-year-old male child

CC: Fever & vomiting
The child is autistic. He has a lack of an appetite and he vomited once yesterday. There is a subjective fever and he complains of a headache; his temperature has not been taken.
Disposition: The mother is advised to take his temperature and give him Children's Motrin (100mg/5mL, 2 teaspoons every 6-8 hours) or Children's Tylenol (160mg/5mL, 2 teaspoons every 4-6 hours) for fever (temperature ≥100.4°F [38.0°C]). She is to offer fluids (juice, soup, ginger ale), and to observe. He may be checked tomorrow.

## Case #457

Autumn                                                    Time: 9:20PM

A three-year-old female child

CC: Head injury
The child slipped from the sofa and hit her head on the coffee table. She cried immediately, and she had no loss of consciousness, nor vomiting, nor any other problem. The mother has applied an ice pack on the child's head.
Disposition: She is advised to use an ice pack wrapped in the towel on the child's head 15 minutes per hour for a couple of hours and to observe. She should call us back if the child vomits in succession or is not behaving appropriately and may seek immediate care in those cases.

## Case #458

Autumn                                                    Time: 12:30AM

An eight-month-old female infant

CC: Woke up crying

The mother states that the infant has been fine but she woke up about an hour ago, because of loud music and has been crying a great deal. She is now asleep. The mother is concerned as to why this occurred and wants to know what to do if it happens again. Disposition: The mother is advised to avoid playing loud music around the infant when she is asleep.

## Case #459

Autumn                                                            Time: 7:10AM

A three-week-old female neonate

CC: Constipation
The neonate's temperature is 99.6°F (37.5°C) and she has not had any bowel movements since yesterday; she is otherwise fine.
Disposition: The mother is advised to offer the baby some water to drink and to observe. If the baby looks fine with no vomiting, and she is not cranky and her abdomen is soft, then the neonate is just to be observed. A temperature up to 100.3°F (37.9°C) is considered normal. To help the infant have a bowel movement, the mother may take a rectal thermometer and lubricate the tip of the thermometer with Vaseline and gently take the neonate's rectal temperature. This maneuver often results in a bowel movement.

## Case #460

Autumn                                                            Time: 6:30PM

A one-month-old male neonate

CC: Facial rash
The baby has a facial rash. He is otherwise fine.
Disposition: The mother is advised to observe and see if the rash is related to anything. If she is using soap on the baby's face, then she is to avoid that. If she feels that the rash is related to the cow's milk base formula, then she can change the formula to a soy-based formula and observe. If the rash was related to the formula, then in one or two weeks she may see an improvement. Breastfed infants might show a reaction to one of the components of the maternal breastmilk, and in this case, she should refrain from eating hyper-allergenic foods and drinking too much cow's milk and observe. Often, a facial rash might just be neonatal acne for which there is little to do.

## CASE #461

AUTUMN                                                    TIME: 9:30PM

A two-month-old male infant

CC: Flatulence

The infant has been straining and passing gas.

Disposition: The mother is asked about the baby's formula and breastmilk consumption. A cow's milk based formula may cause gas. If breastfed, then the mother should avoid consumption of cow's milk or gas producing foods like onions, radishes, cauliflower and beans. The Lactofree formulas or soy formulas have no lactose and could be tolerated better when the infant is colicky and has a great deal of flatulence. It can be normal for infants to strain. Simethicone drops are also helpful for flatulence.

## CASE #462

AUTUMN                                                    TIME: 10:30PM

An eleven-month-old male infant

CC: Eye discharge

The infant has been having eye discharge since about 2 weeks ago, he was checked but no eye drops were given. The child had a similar episode in the past and the mother had been using Sulfacetamide ophthalmic drops previously and now had a question as to whether she may just use those drops.

Disposition: The mother is advised not to use the previous eye drops until the physician checks the eyes and advises her. The mother is also advised regarding the eye hygiene (to clean the eyes with sterile water) and the infant is to be reexamined, an eye culture may be taken if required and appropriate eye drops are to be prescribed if need be. Additionally, the child's ears will be checked, as eye infections often occur concomitantly with ear infection.

## CASE #463

AUTUMN                                                    TIME: 11:20PM

A ten-month-old male infant

CC: Cough

The infant has had a cough for two days. He has had no history of asthma. His temperature is taken via his axilla and is 99.7ºF (37.6ºC).

Disposition: The mother is advised to offer him fluids (juice, soup, and water), she may use a humidifier in the room, and she is to observe him. She is to have the infant examined tomorrow if he is not improving.

## Case #464

AUTUMN                                                    Time: 11:35PM

A three-year-old male toddler

CC: Constipation

The child has been constipated for two days, and has no other problems. He is asleep now.

Disposition: The mother is advised regarding constipation, diet, and bowel regulation. She is advised to cut down on starchy foods in his diet. Increase the amount of fluids (water, juices like prune, apricot, pear or peach) and fibers (oatmeal cereal, fruits and vegetables). She may also try a tablespoon of mineral oil and observe.

## Case #465

AUTUMN                                                    Time: 11:45PM

A three-year-old female child

CC: Fever & an earache

The child has temperature of 101.0ºF (38.3ºC) and she has an earache. She was seen by a physician 2-3 days ago, and has been on Amoxicillin.

Disposition: The mother is advised that if the child has a fever and is cranky, then she should be reexamined.

The pathogen may be resistant to Amoxicillin, as the child has been taking the Amoxicillin for 2-3 days and still has the problem.

Amoxicillin should be given (80-90mg/kg body weight per day, divided in 2-3 doses) for the treatment of acute otitis media. However, if the child is on an appropriate dose and is not responding, then the antibiotic should be changed.

## Case #466

AUTUMN                                                    Time: 3:45AM

A four-year-old male child

CC: Cough & fever

The child has been coughing and has a temperature of 101.8°F (38.7°C). He has received ibuprofen and albuterol. The child had been seen by a physician 2 days ago, and diphenhydramine syrup (Benadryl), albuterol, and ibuprofen were advised. Now the child is coughing a great deal.

Disposition: The mother is advised to use the albuterol MDI, 2 puffs via spacer and she may repeat it in 20 minutes if he is still coughing at that time. If the child is coughing a great deal, then the albuterol may even be repeated twice (after 20 minutes). She is to offer him more fluids (water, Gatorade, ginger ale) and is to continue the albuterol MDI via spacer 2 puffs every 4 hours for 5 days and then every 6 hours for 5 days more. For the fever, a temperature of 100.4°F (38.0°C) or more, she may give him ibuprofen (Children's Motrin 100 mg/5mL, 6 mL every 6-8 hours). If he continues to have a fever or he is in any distress, then he is to be examined in the ED.

When the asthmatic patient is on diphenhydramine (an antihistamine), he or she should be well hydrated. Otherwise, dryness of the mucous membranes, which is a side effect of antihistamine, may exacerbate the asthma.

## Case #467

Autumn                                              Time; 4:30AM

A 14-month-old female infant

CC: Fever

The child has had a temperature of 101.6°F (38.6°C) today. Acetaminophen has been given, and the temperature is down. The mother would like to know what she should do.

Disposition: The mother is advised regarding the temperature; if it comes back and other symptoms associated with fever like cold symptoms, bowel problems, or a skin rash, etc. appear; then she is to take the infant to be checked at the clinic later today. If the fever remains below 102.2°F (39.0°C), then she may continue to observe him at home, as low-grade fevers (below 102.2°F [39.0°C]) may accompany teething symptoms.

## Case #468

Winter                                              Time: 6:42PM

A four-month-old female infant

CC: Fever
The infant has a fever; her temperature is 103.6ºF (39.7ºC). Her mother has been giving her Tylenol but the infant continues to have a fever.
Disposition: The mother is advised to take the infant to be checked at the ED tonight. A young infant with a high fever should be checked early.

## Case #469
Winter                                                    Time: 7:10PM

A two-month-old male infant

CC: Eczema
The infant has eczema.
Disposition: The mother is asked about the infant's formula. A cow's milk based formula may be contributing or may even be the cause of the eczema. If breastfed, and the mom consumes the cow's milk, then the proteins from the milk she is consuming may be contributory, so she may avoid cow's milk in her diet. The use of topical soaps or lotions and laundry detergents used to wash infant's clothing, etc. all should be considered as potential contributors and potentially changing these to mild agents like Dove Sensitive soap or Dreft detergent, for example, may be helpful.
The mother is also advised to take the infant to the clinic tomorrow, so that the infant may be examined and given appropriate cream or ointment if required.

## Case #470
Winter                                                    Time: 7:47PM

A ten-year-old female child

CC: Dysuria & abdominal pain
The child is complaining of pain in her left lower abdomen and she has a low-grade fever. She also complains when urinating. She has had no vomiting and no constipation.
Disposition: The mother is advised to take her to be checked tonight. The child has dysuria, fever, and abdominal pain. She should be examined and have a urinalysis and a urine culture to look for a urinary tract infection.

## Case #471
Winter                                                    Time: 8:37PM

A four-month-old female infant

CC: Fever

The infant has a fever; her temperature is 101.2°F (38.4°C). Tylenol was given about two hours ago, but she still has a fever and she has been cranky. Her appetite is less than usual and she has had no bowel movement today.

Disposition: The mother is advised to take the infant to be checked.

A 4-month-old infant with fever and crankiness should be examined early on, to make sure she does not have a urinary tract infection or other bacterial infection; a work-up is to be done and the infant is to receive appropriate treatments.

## CASE #472
WINTER                                                    TIME: 11:26PM

A one-month-old male neonate

CC: Flatulence

The mother states that the baby has too much gas after taking his formula. He is on Enfamil with iron.

Disposition: The mother is advised to change the formula to a lactose-free (Lactofree) formula and observe whether this measure helps.

## CASE #473
WINTER                                                    TIME: 12:05AM

A ten-month-old male infant

CC: Cold symptoms & spitting up

The infant has a cold and spits up the milk.

Disposition: The mother is advised to use Normal Saline nose drops (1-2 drops into the nostrils, three or four times per day for 3-5 days) and to give him clear fluids (water, white grape juice, broth, Pedialyte), to use a humidifier around him, and to observe. He may be checked in the morning if need be.

## CASE #474
LATE WINTER                                               TIME: 4:46PM

A 17-year-old male adolescent

CC: Question about receiving Gamma globulin.

The adolescent has question regarding his Intravenous Gamma globulin; he has not received his monthly injection of Gamma globulin this month as yet.

Disposition: He is advised to call back tomorrow morning to receive it. He is receiving monthly Gamma globulin because of a serum immune deficiency.

## CASE #475

LATE WINTER                                                    TIME: 7:40PM

A ten-month-old male infant

CC: Question about medication

The mother wanted to know the dose of Pediacare for the cold.

The mother could not be connected via the operator, because she was not available. For the cold symptoms in infants, Normal Saline nose drops/spray are a safe and effective medication to be used for a few days to wash out the mucous membrane of the nasopharynx. Pediacare Children's Decongestant contains a sympathomimetic, Phenylephrine HCL and so is not recommended for infants and children below 6 years of age.

## CASE #476

LATE WINTER                                                    TIME: 7:46PM

A four-month-old male infant

CC: Diarrhea & vomiting

The infant has diarrhea and has vomited two times today. He has no fever; there is neither blood nor mucus in his stool, no bile and no blood in the vomitus. He has been urinating well.

Disposition: The mother is advised to start Pedialyte, by giving him small amounts and making sure he can retain the Pedialyte. If he cannot keep the Pedialyte down, he is to be seen at the ED. Otherwise, she may continue the Pedialyte for a few feedings, then give him lactose-free formula and have him checked tomorrow if required.

## CASE #477

LATE WINTER                                                    TIME: 10:21PM

A four-year-old male child

CC: Nose trauma

The child hit his nose yesterday. He had some nose bleeding at that time and a scrape on his nose.

Today he has some swelling and a bruise on the left side of his nose and under his left eye. Disposition: The mother is advised to apply an ice pack (wrapped in the towel, applied for 15 minutes every hour) onto the swelling. If the swelling appears severe or if he is uncomfortable, then she is to take the child to be checked tonight.

## CASE #478
SPRING                                                           TIME: 5:35PM

A one-month-old female neonate

CC: Vomiting

The neonate has been vomiting since yesterday.

Disposition: The mother is advised to offer the baby Pedialyte and take the baby to be checked.

A one-month-old neonate with vomiting should be checked soon.

## CASE #479
SPRING                                                           TIME: 8:35PM

A 16-month-old male infant

CC: Head trauma

The mother states that the child fell and hit his head on the carpeted floor. He had no loss of consciousness and he is fine. The mother wants to know the dose of Tylenol.

Disposition: The mother is advised that the baby may be given 10-15mg/kg of body weight of Tylenol per dose, which for this child is 80mg of Infants' Tylenol. Tylenol may be given every 4-6 hours as needed for pain. She can also apply an ice pack (wrapped in the towel) to the child's head.

## CASE #480
SPRING                                                           TIME: 9:27PM

A 14-month-old female infant

CC: Reaction to apple juice

The child developed loose bowel movements and some hives after drinking apple juice. She is breathing well and is otherwise well.

Disposition: The mother is advised to avoid giving her apple juice. She may give her 2mL of Benadryl syrup (12.5mg/5mL) every 6 hours for the hives and keep her on a bland diet (Pedialyte, ginger ale, rice cereal, banana and plain yogurt) for diarrhea until she improves.

## Case #481

Spring                                                                    Time: 7:25AM

An eight-year-old female child

CC: Pinkish urine

The mother states that the child has been having pinkish urine off and on for a while. She is otherwise fine.

Disposition: The mother is advised to have the child checked today and to have a urine test done.

The pinkish urine could be because of hematuria (intact red blood cells in the urine), hemoglobinuria (hemolyzed red cells in the urine), myoglobin, porphyrins and bile pigments (red blood cell components). Also, discoloration from some foods like beets, blackberries, food colorings and high concentrations of vitamin C. Drugs that might cause false positive dipstick reading for blood in the urine are: ibuprofen, sulfamethoxazole, nitrofurantoin, rifampin, phenytoin, L-dopa, quinine, and phenazopyridine (Pyridium).

## Case #482

Spring                                                                    Time: 7:20PM

An eight-month-old male infant

CC: Cold symptoms & watery eyes

The infant has had a cold for 2-3 days. He has watery eyes; his rectal temperature is 98.8°F (37.1°C).

Disposition: The mother is advised to offer him fluids (juice, soup, water, and formula or breastmilk). She is to use Normal Saline nose drops (1-2 drops into the nostrils, three or four times per day for 3-5 days), to use a humidifier, and to observe. The baby should be examined if the cold persists (lasts more than 7-10 days or if the fevers are ≥102.2°F (39.0°C)).

# Case #483

Spring                                                              Time: 8:30PM

A two-week-old female neonate

CC: Lump
The mother has felt a small lump in the inner part of her left arm. She has neither fever nor tenderness, and no other problem.
Disposition: The mother is advised to take her to be checked tomorrow.

# Case #484

Spring                                                              Time: 10:09PM

An eleven-year-old male child

CC: Reaction to soy
The child has been vomiting about six or seven times following having eaten some sunflower seeds which had some soy oil and the child is allergic to soy. His mother used his EpiPen and gave him an injection, and has since offered him ginger ale. He currently feels better (back to baseline).
Disposition: The mother is advised to offer him Pedialyte in small amounts frequently, to make sure he can retain it, and to observe him. The child who has been vomiting several times needs fluid with electrolytes. Pedialyte and Gatorade are fluids that help to replenish lost electrolytes.

# Case #485

Winter                                                             Time: 6:14PM

A two-year-old female child

CC: Constipation
The child has had constipation. She has not had any bowel movements for two days. Today, she did have one, however it was hard and there was slight blood from her anal area.
Disposition: The mother is advised to offer her juices like prune or pear juice, give her oatmeal instead of rice cereal, avoid starchy foods and incorporate some vegetables and fruits into her diet. She can also reduce the number of dairy products she consumes. She may also give her a tablespoon of mineral oil. The mother is advised to keep the

child's anal area clean, wash the area with warm water, and to observe.

## Case #486

A seven-year-old female child

CC: Streptococcal pharyngitis & rash

The child had a strep throat infection and received a penicillin injection. She has developed a slightly itchy rash.

Disposition: The mother is advised to give her one teaspoon of Benadryl (12.5mg/5mL) and observe her.

Benadryl, the antihistamine diphenhydramine HCL, 5mg/kg per day in 4 divided doses is used for allergic conditions. The mildly itchy rash might be related to the streptococcal infection as well.

## Case #487

A two-month-old female infant

CC: Question about the dose of Tylenol

The infant received her immunizations today. She has a fever and her mother would like to know how much Tylenol she can give her. She is otherwise well.

Disposition: The mother is advised to give her 40 mg of Infants' Tylenol for fever and that this may be given every 4 to 6 hours for temperatures $\geq 100.4°F$ ($38.0°C$).

## Case #488

A 15-month-old female infant

CC: Rash

The child has a rash and a runny nose; she has no fever. The mother states that she noticed the rash yesterday and that it is itchy. The child has no history of allergy. The mother would like to know if she can give her Benadryl.

Disposition: The mother is advised that she may give her 2mL of Benadryl syrup (12.5mg/5mL) every 6 hours if she has an itchy rash and to observe the baby. Benadryl is antihistamine, diphenhydramine HCL, and is indicated for allergic disorders. The dose for children is 5mg/kg per day in 4 divided doses.

## Case #489

An 11-month-old male infant

CC: Burn
The infant had burn on his arm 2-3 nights ago, for which he has been seen. Today when the mother was changing the burn dressing, she noted one or two spots of blood. Disposition: The mother is advised to keep the wound clean and to continue to use the proper ointment like Silvadine or Bacitracin and to continue the dressing changes. She is to have the child checked in the clinic.

## Case #490

A 16-month-old male infant

CC: Medication refill request
The child had a prescription for Phenobarbital but the amount of the medicine was not written on the prescription; Phenobarbital is a controlled medicine and the pharmacist needs to know the exact amount to dispense. I advised him to give them small amount to use over the weekend but the pharmacist refused.
The pharmacist was advised to call the prescribing physician directly to get the complete prescription information.

## Case #491

A ten-day-old female neonate

CC: Breastfeeding/feeding schedule
The mother had a question regarding breastfeeding.
Disposition: The mother was advised and explained how often she should breastfeed the baby. Initially the baby should feed on demand, then she may gradually extend the time between two feedings to every 3 hours, and later every 4 hours.

# Case #492

Time: 3:18PM

A three-year-old female child

CC: Stomatitis (infection of the mouth)
The child complains that her mouth hurts.
Disposition: The mother is advised to give her mild and soft foods, rinse her mouth with cool water after she eats, and to observe the child. She should make sure the child drinks enough fluid. She may be checked in the clinic tomorrow.

# Case #493

Winter                                                    Time: 4:07PM

A one-month-old female infant

CC: Loose bowel movements
The mother states that the baby had about 2 ounces of cow's milk instead of her formula yesterday and that she has had several small loose bowel movements today. The infant looks well otherwise.
Disposition: The mother is advised to give her Pedialyte (instead of formula) for one or two feedings. She is then to resume giving her formula. She is to avoid feeding her cow's milk. Cow's milk is not recommended for infants bellow one year of age. If the infant looks dehydrated (dry mucous membranes, not voiding every 6 hours), then she is to have her checked at the ED.

# Case #494

Winter                                                    Time: 9:26PM

A nine-month-old male infant

CC: Cold symptoms
The infant has a cold; his axillary temperature is 99.8°F (37.6°C) and he has been shivering. He has had neither vomiting nor diarrhea.
Disposition: The mother is advised to give him 80mg of Infants' Tylenol for a rectal temperature ≥100.4°F (38.0°C). She is to offer him fluids (juice, soup, flat ginger ale) to drink and observe. If he drinks fluids well, has no vomiting, and is well-appearing, then he may be checked tomorrow morning.

## CASE #495

TIME: 10:15PM

An eleven-month-old male infant

CC: Itchy eyes

The father states that the infant rubs his eyes. There is a red spot on the upper eyelid of one of his eyes. He may have a low-grade fever.

Disposition: The father is advised regarding eye hygiene (clean the eyes with sterile water) and giving him acetaminophen for fever.

The infant likely has an insect bite or a stye on the eyelid. He may be observed and if worsening or not improving, he can be seen in the clinic.

## CASE #496

WINTER                                                     TIME: 11:58PM

A one-year-old male infant

CC: Cough/asthma

The child has been coughing and he has a history of asthma. The mother states that the child is coughing a great deal; he has received his asthma treatment via nebulizer but he is still coughing.

Disposition: The mother is advised to repeat the treatment (albuterol) in 20 minutes, give him one teaspoon of prednisolone (Orapred15mg/5ml) syrup, and observe. If he vomits, is in any distress, or is not improving, then he is to be seen at the ED. If his cough is much better after the steroids and the second treatment, then she may continue to give the albuterol via nebulizer every 4 hours for 4-5 days, then every 6 hours until he has no cough. She can continue to give the prednisolone syrup for 3-5 days, and she is to keep his appointment for asthma follow-up.

## CASE #497

WINTER                                                     TIME: 3:45AM

A 23-month-old male infant

CC: Blister in the mouth

The mother states that the child had blisters in his mouth and was seen at the hospital four days ago. He has been drinking juice and eating yogurt. He had a normal bowel movement yesterday afternoon. He vomited the juice last night. The mother states that he vomited bile (dark green vomit).

Disposition: The mother is advised that if he vomited bile or he is fussy, then he should be seen at the ED.

Vomiting bile is a sign of gastrointestinal tract obstruction and so the toddler should be checked immediately.

## Case #498

Winter                                                                          Time: 8:45PM

A six-month-old female infant

CC: Cold symptoms & cough
The infant has cold symptoms, a cough, and no fever.

Disposition: The mother is advised to use Normal Saline nose drops (1-2 drops into the nostrils three or four times per day for 3-5 days), to offer her fluids (water, juice, and formula or breastmilk), to use a humidifier in the room, and to observe. She may be examined at the clinic tomorrow.

## Case #499

Spring                                                                          Time: 4:47PM

A 17-year-old female adolescent

CC: Question about HPV
The teenager was seen at the clinic today and she was concerned about HPV.

Disposition: The adolescent is advised that HPV (human papillomavirus) infection, has a viral origin and is transmitted by close contact, person to person, and causes warts on the skin and affects the genitalia. Symptomatic individuals should be checked and treated. It is the most common sexually transmitted infection. There are different types of HPV viruses, and the type of the HPV virus can be determined, since some types of HPV virus require more attention. She is advised to make an appointment to be checked at the adolescent clinic.

HPV (human papillomaviruses) are DNA viruses and there are cutaneous and mucosal types. Among the high risk mucosal types, type 16 and type 18 are associated with cervical cancer. Protection against these strains are included in the available HPV vaccines.

HPV vaccines have been available for over a decade now for the prevention of genital warts, cervical and anal cancers in females. The vaccines also protect males from genital warts, penile cancers and anal cancers. They are also likely to protect against some oropharyngeal cancers (cancers of the throat, tonsils, base of the tongue, soft palate). HPV vaccines are not live virus vaccines and so can be given to immunocompromised persons including those afflicted with infection (HIV), or those on immunosuppressive medications.

## CASE #500

SPRING                                                    TIME: 6:08PM

A seven-year-old male child

CC: Question about the medication

The child was just started on Ritalin 5mg tablets. He will be taking his first dose tomorrow morning. He is also on Amoxicillin. The mother would like to know if it is okay to take the Ritalin while he is on Amoxicillin.

Disposition: The mother is advised that the child may take both medications simultaneously.

There are no interactions between Ritalin (the stimulant, methylphenidate HCL) and Amoxicillin.

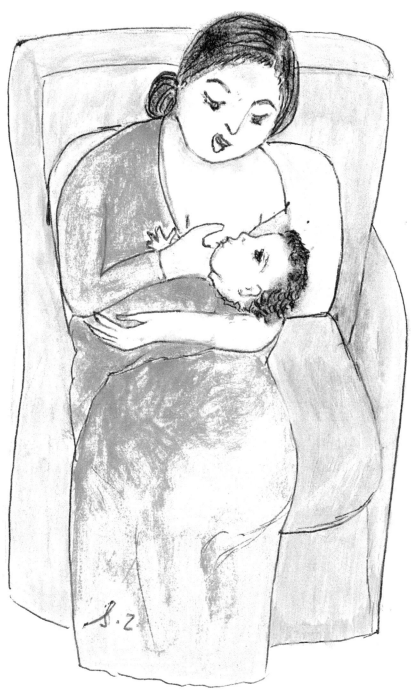

A Case of Breastfeeding infant

# CHAPTER ELEVEN

~~~

## CASE #501

A nine-month-old male infant

CC: Fever
The infant started having a fever today. The mother states that the infant was given 80mg of Infants' Tylenol an hour ago, and that his temperature is currently 102.8°F (39.3°C).
Disposition: The mother is advised to take the infant to be checked at the ED.
An infant with a persistent fever should be checked. If the temperature is ≥102.2°F (39.0°C) in a child less than 3 year of age, then the child should be examined.


## CASE #502

SPRING                                                    TIME: 8:39PM

A two-year-old female toddler

CC: Strep throat, febrile seizure, & leg movements
The child has had a fever concomitant with a seizure two days ago. She was seen at the hospital and a throat swab revealed a Streptococcal infection for which she received a penicillin injection. Also, there was further laboratory testing done and an EEG (electroencephalogram) is to be done later. The child has been having a hard time falling asleep and she has been having leg movements.
Disposition: A child with persistent fevers and with abnormal involuntary movements

should be reevaluated. While this child appears to have febrile seizures, the new leg movements should be evaluated. The mother is also advised to treat the child's fever if it persists, and to get in touch with her pediatrician to arrange for the EEG.

## Case #503

Spring                                                                     Time: 7:59AM

A four-year-old male child

CC: Red, swollen eyes
The child woke up with red and swollen eyes today. The mother denies any other problems.
Disposition: The mother is advised to apply a sterile cold compress on the eyes for about 5 minutes every hour and to have the child checked today.
In the springtime, allergic conjunctivitis is prevalent due to the pollens of the flowers and trees in the air. The child should be checked and given appropriate treatment.

## Case #504

Spring                                                                     Time: 7:08AM

An eight-month-old male infant

CC: Fever
The infant has been having a fever since yesterday. He was just examined by his pediatrician yesterday at his well-baby check-up and Tylenol was advised. He was not given any vaccines. Today he currently has a temperature of 102.0°F (38.8°C), and no medicine has been given for the fever.
Disposition: The mother is advised to give him 80mg of Infants' Tylenol for fever, which she can continue to administer every 4-6 hours for temperatures ≥100.4°F (38.0°C). She should also offer him fluids (water, juice, and formula or breast milk) and observe. If he were to develop a temperature above 102.2°F (39.0°C), then she is to take the infant to be rechecked.

## Case #505

Spring                                                                     Time: 8:30PM

A two-year-old male child

CC: Cold symptoms

The child has been having a temperature of 100.0°F (37.7°C) during the last four days. The father states that he had vomited on the first day of his illness; there was no blood nor bile in the vomitus. He was offered clear fluids like juice and Gatorade. He is no longer vomiting, but now he has a stuffy nose, runny nose, and a slight cough.

Disposition: The father is advised to use Normal Saline nose drops (1-2 drops into the nostrils, 3-4 times per day for 3-5 days) and to use a humidifier in the room. For temperatures ≥100.4°F (38.0°C), he may give him 160mg of Children's Tylenol (160mg/5mL, one teaspoon every 4-6 hours). Also, the father is advised to offer him fluids (juice, soup, ginger ale) and observe. If the child were to develop a fever ≥102.2°F (39.0°C), then he may be checked at that point.

## Case #506

Spring                                                     Time: 3:54AM

An eight-month-old male infant

CC: High fever

The infant has a fever; his temperature is 103.4°F (39.6°C). He has been drinking well and acting normally. He was given 80mg of Infants' Tylenol. He has been having a fever for 3 days and is otherwise fine.

Disposition: The mother is advised regarding Roseola, a viral infection that causes high fever for 3-4 days with a well appearing child. When the fever resolves, a rash will appear on the trunk. If the infant is cranky, has vomiting, or looks sick, then he is to be checked at the ED. Otherwise, she may have him checked in the morning at the clinic. After the age of 6 months, Motrin (ibuprofen) may also be given to help control high temperature.

Human herpesvirus-6 (HHV-6) is responsible virus for Roseola infantum infection. Roseola is more prevalent in infants and young children between the ages of 6 months to 3 years.

## Case #507

Spring                                                     Time: 10:48AM

A two-year-old male toddler

CC: Medication question

The child has an ear infection and is taking an antibiotic. The mother has a question regarding how to give the medicine.

Disposition: The mother is advised on medication administration.

She can measure the medicine with a syringe and put it into the corner of the child's mouth (between the cheek and the gums) and then close his mouth and give him some water or juice (orange juice) to drink just after giving the medicine to help to remove the taste of the medication. It is better not to add the medicine to juice as children often do not finish the juice containing the medication, and so we will not know if they have received the appropriate amount of the medicine. The mother is advised to keep the child's appointment for follow-up.

## Case #508

An eight-month-old female infant

CC: Reaction to Amoxicillin

The infant has a rash. The mother states that the child has been on Amoxicillin for about one week. The infant had developed a rash at the onset of the treatment, but had simultaneously tried canned spaghetti with tomato sauce and mango for the first time. She was seen by her pediatrician and the rash was attributed to the foods and she was advised to continue the Amoxicillin. Now the rash is getting worse. The child does not appear to be bothered by the rash. She is otherwise well without any respiratory concerns and is eating and drinking well.

Disposition: The mother is advised to stop the Amoxicillin, use Calamine lotion on the rash, and to observe. She has an appointment to be checked tomorrow for follow-up. The mother is advised to keep the appointment tomorrow.

## Case #509

A three-year-old male child

CC: Diarrhea with mucus

The child has been having diarrhea with mucus in the stool for one week. He has been seen by a physician, and a stool test was done and the result is pending. He has not had any blood in the stool.

Disposition: The mother is advised to give him more fluids (Pedialyte, white grape juice, ginger ale) and to offer him foods like white rice, applesauce, banana, and plain yogurt; he also can have hard-boiled egg, well-cooked white meat (chicken or turkey breast). She is to avoid giving him milk and dairy products, beans, and raw fruits and vegetables for one or two weeks. She is advised to follow the result of the stool test.

## CASE #510
EARLY SUMMER                                                    TIME: 8:37PM

A two-year-old female toddler

CC: Cough
The child has been having a cough for three days. She has not had any fever. The child has no history of asthma and has had no wheezing.
Disposition: The mother is advised to offer her fluids (water, juice, soup, ginger ale), and to use Normal Saline nose drops into her nostrils (1-2 drops, 3-4 times per day for 3-5 days) to wash out the mucous membranes of the nasopharynx and help clear the virus or allergen. She may also use a humidifier in the room and observe. If the cough is frequent, if the toddler develops a fever, or if the cold lasts longer than 5-7 days, then she should have the toddler examined.

## CASE #511
EARLY SUMMER                                                    TIME: 9:16PM

A four-month-old female infant

CC: Post-immunization fever
The infant had her immunizations today and currently has a slight fever. She is otherwise well, feeding well, and is not fussy.
Disposition: The father is advised that having a fever following immunizations is a common side effect. He can give her 40mg of Infants' Tylenol every 4-6 hours for fever and observe. If the fever were to be ≥102.2°F (39.0°C) following immunizations, or if the fever were to last more than 2 days, then the baby would need to be checked.

## CASE #512
EARLY SUMMER                                                    TIME: 9:47PM

A three-year-old male child

CC: Pica (chewing/eating non-food items/things with no nutritional value)

The mother noticed paint in the child's mouth. She rinsed the mouth and called the poison control center. She was told that the paint is nontoxic.

Disposition: The mother is advised regarding prevention and the child to be observed. A child that puts non-food substances in the mouth has Pica. The mother should make an appointment with the Pediatrician and when seen, should have a blood test for anemia and a lead test.

A blood lead level of ≥10mcg/dL is elevated and is of concern. Iron deficiency enhances the absorption of lead in the guts; therefore, the blood test for anemia should be done concomitantly and iron deficiency is to be treated.


# Case #513

Early summer                                                    Time: 11:14PM

A nine-day-old male neonate

CC: Constipation

The father thinks that the baby is constipated. His last bowel movements had been last night. He is presently asleep and comfortable. The bowel movements have been of normal consistency (yellow, seedy, mustard-like).

Disposition: The father is advised regarding the feeding and bowel movements. He can offer him small amount of boiled and then cooled water and observe, massage his belly, bicycle his legs and gently take a rectal temperature. Sometimes an infant might not pass stool daily, and if the neonate is comfortable, his abdomen is soft and he is not vomiting, it is acceptable just to observe him and make sure he is taking an adequate amount of formula or breastmilk.


# Case #514

Summer                                                          Time: 8:39PM

A three-year-old male toddler

CC: Fever, rash, & mouth lesions

The child has a fever, a rash, and some blisters on his tongue.

Disposition: The mother is advised regarding the viral condition. She is to offer the child mild and soft foods (baby foods, applesauce, Jell-O and ice cream) and fluids (water, white grape juice, Gatorade), give him Children's Tylenol (160mg/5mL, one teaspoon every 4-6 hours) for fever, and to observe.

The responsible viruses are enteroviruses like coxsackievirus and echoviruses. The prevalence is mostly in the summer and fall.

## CASE #515

TIME: 10:49PM

A four-month-old male infant

CC: Post-immunization fever
The infant has a fever; his temperature is 101.0°F (38.3°C). He was given his immunizations today. The father has given him Infants' Tylenol for his fever. He has been taking his formula well.
Disposition: The father is advised that the infant may continue to have Infants' Tylenol (40mg every 4-6 hours) for temperatures ≥100.4°F (38.0°C). He may also be offered cool water to drink, when he has a fever. If the temperature is ≥102.2°F (39.0°C) after immunizations or if the fever lasts longer than 2 days after the immunizations, then the child should be checked.

## CASE #516

SUMMER TIME: 12:16AM

An eleven-month-old male infant

CC: Febrile Seizure
The infant has a fever; his temperature is 102.5°F (39.1°C). He had a febrile seizure for about a few seconds. Motrin has been given for the fever. The mother is asking for the dose of Children's Motrin.
Disposition: The mother is advised regarding the dose of Children's Motrin (100mg/5mL) oral suspension. For temperatures ≥100.4°F (38.0°C) he may be given one teaspoon of Children's Motrin oral suspension (10mg per kg body weight per dose) every 6 to 8 hours. The mother is also advised to offer the infant more fluid to drink whenever he has a fever. She should take him to the ED to be checked now.

## CASE #517

SUMMER TIME: 6:43PM

A four-day-old female neonate

CC: Breastfeeding

The baby is breastfeeding; her mother has a breast problem. She is taking a medication. She was told that she could continue to breastfeed the baby, as it would be safe for the baby. She is asking if she can feed the baby formula for a few days instead of breastfeeding.

Disposition: The mother is advised regarding the advantages of breastfeeding, including the transfer of antibodies that the baby receives through the breastmilk. She is also told that the composition of the breastmilk facilitates the absorption of iron and that breastmilk is easily digested. She is told that breastfeeding facilitates bonding between the neonate and the mother. She is also advised on how to extract her milk using the breast-pump regularly, and that she is to drink more fluid to increase her milk supply. She is to have good breast and nipple hygiene. She should breastfeed the infant just before taking her medicine, and she can also give the baby some formula in between if she has some difficulties secondary to her breast condition, or due to the medicine she is taking. She may resume breastfeeding as soon as her breast problem is improving.

## CASE #518

SUMMER                                                                    TIME: 12:18AM

A five-month-old female infant

CC: Fever

The infant has a fever; her temperature is currently 101.0°F (38.3°C). She has no other problems.

Disposition: The mother is advised to give her 40mg of Infants' Tylenol for fever, offer her more fluids (water, white grape juice, and formula or breastmilk), and to observe the baby. If the fever persists or is ≥102.2°F (39.0°C), then she is to be checked.

## CASE #519

SUMMER                                                                     TIME: 2:13AM

A 12-year-old male child

CC: Prepuce (foreskin of the penis) bleeding

The mother states that the child says there was bleeding when the prepuce was pulled back.

Disposition: The mother is advised to wash and dry the affected area on the child's prepuce. He may use baby shampoo to wash the area and may use some Bacitracin (antibiotic) ointment on it, twice a day. If he has any problems when he is urinating because of the tight prepuce (phimosis), then he is to be checked.

## Case #520

Summer                                                                                    Time: 7:44PM

An eight-month-old female infant

CC: Not eating well

The mother had told the answering service that the baby was not eating well. There was no response when I called her.

If the infant truly has a poor appetite, then she should be checked at the clinic and have a blood test for anemia (CBC [complete blood count], looking at the Hgb [hemoglobin] and HCT [hematocrit], and a lead test). Iron deficiency anemia can cause a poor appetite. An elevated blood lead level has inhibiting effects in the heme pathway in the cells and competes with iron and so causes iron deficiency anemia. Treatment of iron deficiency anemia (with elemental iron 3-6mg/kg of body weight per day) will improve the appetite. The Hgb will be repeated in one month. The iron therapy should be continued for 8 weeks beyond whenever the Hgb normalizes to replenish the iron stores in the liver.

## Case #521

Summer                                                                                    Time: 9:59PM

A two-month-old male infant

CC: Post-immunization fever

The infant has been cranky and has had a slight fever after having received the immunizations, which were just given earlier today.

Disposition: The mother is advised regarding the common side effect of fever after immunizations. She should give the baby 40mg of Infants' Tylenol every 4-6 hours and observe. Given the child's young age, if the infant is excessively cranky or has a high fever ≥102.2°F (39.0°C) after the immunizations, then the infant should be checked. Likewise, if the fever after the immunizations lasts for more than 2 days the infant should be checked.

# Case #522

Time: 11:05PM

A 13-day-old female neonate

CC: Spitting up & vomiting

The baby has been vomiting and spitting up after the feedings. Her bowel movements are normal. The mother has been feeding the baby breastmilk and formula frequently. There is neither blood nor phlegm in the vomitus. She is not fussy and has been urinating well. There are no ill contacts.

Disposition: The mother is advised to breastfeed the baby every 3 hours and that if the baby takes the breastmilk well, and the mother has enough breastmilk, she needs not give her formula. She should keep the baby in an upright position for about 20 minutes after the feedings, burp her often, and observe. When the neonate has normal bowel movements, it implies that the baby is receiving enough milk. Spitting up or vomiting after feedings could be because of over-feeding, too frequent feedings, too much movement after the feedings, or if the baby was kept flat just after the feedings. The mother is advised to observe, and to take the neonate to be checked at the clinic to make sure her weight is appropriate.

# Case #523

Summer

Time: 7:18PM

A five-year-old male child

CC: Rash, one week after MMR immunization

The child has a rash on his body. He received his immunizations (DTaP, IPV, HIB, and MMR) seven days ago.

Disposition: The mother is advised that the rash could be related to the MMR immunization and that the child is to be observed. As the MMR immunization contains live attenuated measles virus, there is the possibility of developing a rash like that of mild measles and that is self-limited. With this vaccine, a fever one week afterwards is also a possibility.

# Case #524

Summer

Time: 8:10PM

A five-month-old male infant

CC: Normal but frequent stool, 4 times today

The infant has had 4 bowel movements after having taken barley cereal today. He has no other problems. His stools appear normal and they are not large amounts.

Disposition: The mother is reassured and advised that the increased fiber has caused an increase in stool frequency.

## CASE #525

SUMMER                                                      TIME: 1:43AM

A five-day-old male neonate

CC: Constipation

The newborn baby has not had any bowel movements today. He is fine and is not fussy. The prior bowel movements have been of normal color and consistency. He is currently comfortable and sleeping.

Disposition: The mother is advised regarding the bowel movements. She is to make sure the baby is taking enough breastmilk or formula, and to observe.

The newborn baby might not have a daily bowel movement, but if the baby is feeling well, voiding normally, has a soft belly without any distention, and is not vomiting, then the baby is likely okay.

## CASE#526

EARLY AUTUMN                                               TIME: 8:50PM

A five-year-old male child

CC: Corneal abrasion

The child has a corneal abrasion and has been on ciprofloxacin ophthalmic solution and bacitracin ophthalmic ointment, each has been used three times per day. The child is complaining of a continued burning sensation of the eyes.

Disposition: The mother is advised to call and consult with the ophthalmologist tomorrow as the dose of ciprofloxacin ophthalmic solution 0.3% is usually used more frequently at the onset of treatment.

## CASE #527

EARLY AUTUMN                                               TIME: 9:20PM

A nine-month-old female infant

CC: Skin lesions

The infant has been having some skin lesions on different parts of her body. She has no fever. The tiny blister-like lesions have been present for 3 days and appear to be mosquito bites.

Disposition: The mother is advised to use Calamine lotion and Bacitracin ointment on the lesions and to have her checked tomorrow.

Molluscum contagiosum is a benign viral condition with no systemic manifestations. The lesions are 2-4 mm diameter dome-shaped papules that are usually pinkish or flesh-colored and central umbilication may be present. About 5-15 discrete papules on the trunk, face and extremities are usually present. It is a self-limited condition and usually resolves spontaneously in 6-12 months, sometimes longer.


## CASE #528

EARLY AUTUMN                                                    TIME: 9:45PM

An 18-month-old male toddler

CC: Head injury

The little boy was running when he tripped and fell and hit his forehead on the floor. He cried immediately and there was no loss of consciousness. There is no bruising.

Disposition: The mother is advised to apply an ice pack wrapped in a towel onto the area that was hit and to observe. If he is acting normally, feels okay, and has no repeated vomiting, then he need not be seen in the ED.


## CASE #529

AUTUMN                                                         TIME: 4:16AM

A two-month-old male infant

CC: Nasal congestion

The infant has nasal congestion and no other problems.

Disposition: The mother is advised to use Normal Saline nose drops 1-2 drops in his nostrils (three times per day for 3-5 days), to use a humidifier around the baby, and to observe.


## CASE #530

AUTUMN                                                         TIME: 7:30AM

A three-year-old female toddler

CC: Fever & a medication question
The child has a fever and the mother would like to know how much Tylenol (acetaminophen) she can give her.
Disposition: The mother is advised to give her one teaspoon of acetaminophen, Children's Tylenol (160mg/5mL), every 4-6 hours for temperatures ≥100.4°F (38.0°C). The mother is advised to have the toddler checked should the fever persist, or if the temperature is ≥102.2°F (39.0°C).

## CASE#531
AUTUMN                                                    TIME: 11:07PM

A six-month-old male infant

CC: Slight cough & some noisy breathing
The infant has a slight cough and was wheezing. He is now sleeping comfortably and appears to be fine.
Disposition: The mother is advised that if the infant has wheezing, vomiting, or any difficulty breathing then she is to take him to the ED tonight to be examined and receive treatment. Otherwise, if he just has a slight cough and is sleeping well without wheezing, then he is to be seen tomorrow morning.

## CASE #532
AUTUMN                                                    TIME: 11:55PM

A six-month-old female infant

CC: Vomiting
The infant has been vomiting. She had been sick last week with a viral infection which resolved recently. About 7 hours ago, while at daycare, she had a jar of carrots and soon after, she vomited. Her mother then offered her 5-6 oz. of Pedialyte, but she also vomited the Pedialyte. There was no blood nor bile in the vomitus. She has had no fever.
Disposition: The mother is advised to try offering the Pedialyte in small amounts (5 mL with a syringe or 1 teaspoon, every minute for 12 minutes) and to observe. If the infant cannot retain the Pedialyte in this fashion, then she is to be checked at the ED.

# Case #533

Time: 1:22AM

A seven-year-old male child

CC: Stomachache & vomiting

The child has a stomachache and has been vomiting. While he was sleeping, he began to have abdominal pains, woke up shaking and vomited twice. He had been having normal bowel movements prior to this. There is neither blood nor bile in the vomitus.

Disposition: The father is advised that he may offer him Pedialyte but that if his pain is severe, if cannot retain the Pedialyte, or if he is ill-appearing, then he should be examined at the ED.

# Case #534

Autumn                                                              Time: 8:10AM

A two-year-old male toddler

CC: Poor appetite

The child is refusing to eat. He has been having a cold for almost one month with a runny nose.

Disposition: The mother is advised regarding runny noses and lack of appetite. The child should be checked by his pediatrician. The mother is to offer him fluids and multivitamin drops (Poly-Vi-Sol 1 mL daily). The physician will make sure he has no secondary infection and he has no iron deficiency anemia, which can cause a lack of appetite. The child may then be treated appropriately if need be.

# Case #535

Autumn                                                              Time: 2:00AM

An eight-month-old male infant

CC: Diarrhea

The infant has been having diarrhea for 2 days. He has neither fever nor vomiting. There is no blood and no mucus in the stool. He is urinating well. The diarrhea began after the infant was given chicken.

Disposition: The mother is advised to offer the infant Pedialyte. The infant is breastfed.

The mother may continue to breastfeed and observe. He may be checked in the clinic later today.

## CASE #536

AUTUMN                                                    TIME: 8:00PM

A four-year-old female child

CC: Cold symptoms

The child has a cold and some nasal congestion. She has no fever.

Disposition: The mother is advised regarding using Normal Saline nose drops 1-2 drops into the nostrils, three or four times per day for 3-5 days and offering her fluids (juice, soup, ginger ale) to drink. She may also use a humidifier in the room and observe.

If the cold lasts longer than 10-12 days, or if she were to develop a fever ≥102.2°F (39.0°C), then the child may be checked at the clinic at that point.

## CASE #537

AUTUMN                                                    TIME: 11:00PM

A four-year-old male child

CC: Fever & vomiting

The child has a fever and has been vomiting. There is no blood and no bile in the vomitus. His bowel movements have been normal and he is urinating well.

Disposition: The mother is advised to take his temperature and give him Children's Tylenol (160mg/5mL, one teaspoon every 4-6 hours) for fever, offer him Pedialyte and clear fluids (white grape juice, ginger ale, Gatorade), and to observe. She is to have him checked at the ED if his temperature is ≥102.2°F (39.0°C), or if the temperature does not respond to Tylenol administration, or if he cannot retain the fluids.

## CASE #538

SPRING                                                    TIME: 6:18PM

A nine-year-old male child

CC: Laceration

The child hit his head against a wooden box that was holding a fire extinguisher and he now has a cut on his head and some bleeding.

Disposition: The mother is advised to use a piece of gauze and apply direct pressure onto the site of the bleeding. She is to put an ice pack on it for a few minutes and observe. If he continues to have bleeding from the cut, then he is to be seen at the ED. The mother is to continue to apply pressure if need be. The mother is to take his immunization records with him and make sure he is up-to-date for his DTaP immunizations.

## CASE #539
SPRING                                                                    TIME: 8:40PM

A three-week-old male neonate

CC: Constipation
The baby is constipated. He has had no bowel movements today.
He is fine and has no other problems. He is now sleeping.
Disposition: The mother is advised to offer him some boiled then cooled water to drink and to observe. Newborn infants do not necessarily have daily bowel movements. If the baby is comfortable, not vomiting, and is not cranky, then he is likely okay. The caregiver should make sure the baby has adequate breastmilk or formula and observe.

## CASE #540
SPRING                                                                    TIME: 9:15PM

A three-year-old female toddler

CC: Fever & a headache
The child has a fever; her temperature is 102.0°F (38.8°C), and she is complaining of a headache. She has no vomiting.
Disposition: The mother is advised to give her Children's Motrin (100mg/5mL, 6mL every 6-8 hours) and offer her fluids (water, juice, ginger ale) to drink and to observe. If she feels better, then she may be checked tomorrow morning. However, if she continues to have a high fever or vomiting, then the mother is to take her to the ED tonight.

## CASE #541
SPRING                                                                    TIME: 11:00PM

A nine-month-old female infant

CC: Vomiting

The infant has had vomiting after the feedings. She has had some yogurt for the first time today. She also had some beef and carrots. There is no blood and no bile in the vomitus. She has had no fever and her bowel movements have been normal. She has been urinating well.

Disposition: The mother is advised to give her Pedialyte and clear fluid (white grape juice) and to observe. She may be checked tomorrow if required.

## CASE#542

SPRING                                                              TIME: 6:38PM

A ten-year-old female child

CC: Loose tooth

Her mother states that the child has a loose tooth on the left lower side of her mouth and that it has been bothering her. The tooth is a baby tooth. She was seen by her dentist yesterday and one of her other teeth were extracted.

Disposition: The mother is advised to give her pain medicine (Tylenol or Motrin) and to increase her oral hygiene (by rinsing her mouth each time after eating by using 8oz. of warm water mixed with a pinch of salt to rinse the mouth). She may be placed on a liquid or soft/mild diet and is to be observed. If despite these measures the symptoms persist, then the mother is to have her checked by the dentist tomorrow.

## CASE #543

SPRING                                                              TIME: 8:31PM

An eight-month-old female infant

CC: Sickle cell disease & a medication question

The infant has sickle cell disease and is on prophylactic penicillin. The mother had a question regarding the dose of the medication.

Disposition: The infant with sickle cell disease should be on prophylactic penicillin at a dose of 125mg twice per day. Once older than age 2, children with sickle cell disease should receive prophylactic penicillin 250mg twice per day.

## CASE #544

SPRING                                                              TIME: 12:45PM

A two-year-old male toddler

CC: Nose injury.
The child was jumping up and down on the bed and hit his nose against the wall. He had slight nose bleeding and no other problems. He has a mark on his nose.
Disposition: The mother is advised to put an ice pack wrapped in a towel on his nose, for 5 to 10 minutes a few times per day, and to observe.


## Case #545

A 13-day-old male neonate

CC: Constipation & straining
The neonate has been constipated and has also been straining.
Disposition: His father is advised regarding normal bowel movements and straining. He is to offer the baby boiled then cooled water to drink and to observe.
Neonates often strain when defecating. This is because some neonates lack coordination between the increased intra-abdominal pressure from the abdominal muscles and the relaxation of the muscles of the pelvic floor at the time of stooling. Infants might not have a daily bowel movement. If the baby is comfortable, the abdomen is soft, and the baby is not vomiting, then the condition could be observed. The caregiver should make sure that the baby has had enough formula or breastmilk. Massaging the belly, bicycling the legs, and gently taking a rectal temperature are other methods that may help an infant have a bowel movement.


## Case #546

A six-month-old female infant

CC: Hoarse voice
The infant has been losing her voice and has been having a hoarse voice today. She has had no fever. She is feeding well.
Disposition: The mother is advised to use a humidifier around the baby and to take her to the bathroom around the steam while the shower is running with warm water. She may be offered warm fluids (warm water, warm formula) to drink and should be observed. She is to be checked if she is in any distress or if the breathing is noisy.

# CASE #547

A one-month-old male neonate

CC: Runny nose & a possible fever
The infant has been having a runny nose; his axillary temperature is 99.0°F (37.2°C). The baby is also fussy, according to his mother.
Disposition: The mother is advised to use Normal Saline nose drops (1-2 drops into the nostrils, three or four times per day for 3-5 days) and to take the temperature rectally. If the temperature is ≥100.4°F (38.0°C), she is to have him examined at the ED. A neonate with fever or fussiness should be checked.

# CASE #548

SPRING                                                               TIME: 5:20PM

A one-month-old female neonate

CC: Conjunctivitis in a neonate
The baby has been having greenish mucus from his eyes for about 2 weeks.
Disposition: The mother is advised to have the baby examined at the ED.
There is the possibility of Chlamydia Trachomatis conjunctivitis in a neonate. A culture from the eye or nonculture method direct fluorescent antibody (DFA) should be used to detect this and the baby is to be treated with erythromycin ethylsuccinate (E.E.S.). Chlamydial eye infection in a neonate should be treated with oral erythromycin, 50mg/kg/day divided into 4 doses for 14 days as topical antibiotics are ineffective.

# CASE #549

SPRING                                                               TIME: 8:49PM

A two-week-old male neonate

CC: Breastfeeding & a question regarding maternal medication
The mother is breastfeeding and has taken some Dulcolax Tablets and some Mylanta. She has been feeding the baby every 2 hours.
She offered the baby 2-3 oz. of formula as a supplement to the breastmilk, and the baby vomited the formula once tonight.
Disposition: The mother is advised to give 2 oz. of clear Pedialyte for one feeding and

to observe. If he has no vomiting, she may resume breastfeeding. If the baby has any problems feeding, then the caregiver is to take the baby to be checked at the ED. Both maternal use of Mylanta and Dulcolax (bisacodyl) are not known to cause any adverse reactions in breastfed infants.

## CASE #550
SPRING                                                    TIME: 10:45PM

An eight-month-old female infant

CC: Exposure to croup
The infant was exposed to croup; she is currently fine.
Disposition: The mother is advised to observe. If the infant develops a hoarse voice, she is to use a humidifier and warm steam around the baby. She may take her into the bathroom where she turns the shower on to create warm steam. She is to offer the baby warm fluids (warm water, warm formula) to drink. If she were to worsen or have noisy breathing at rest, she may be seen in the ED.
Parainfluenza viruses are the major cause of laryngotracheobronchitis (croup). Parainfluenza viruses have different serotypes. Parainfluenza type 3 virus serotype is more prevalent during the spring.

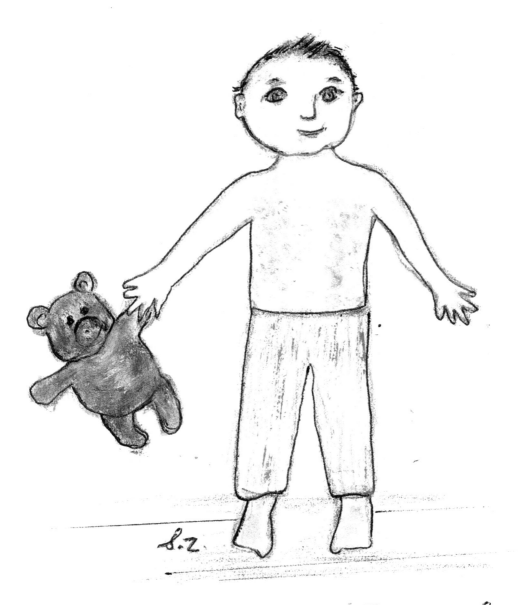

A Toddler with Roseola

# CHAPTER TWELVE

## CASE #551

TIME: 12:01AM

A ten-day-old male neonate

CC: Separation of an extra digit (finger)

The baby was born with an extra digit (finger) which was tied tightly with a string at birth. Now, the mother has noticed that the extra digit has partially separated and that the separated area is red with oozing clear fluid.

Disposition: The mother is advised to clean the skin, apply topical Bacitracin ointment on it, cover it with a piece of sterile gauze, and to observe. If the baby is fussy, has a fever, or if there are signs of infection like redness, warmth, or pain, then she is to have the baby checked at the ED.

## CASE #552

SPRING TIME: 8:04AM

A two-month-old infant

CC: Crankiness

The infant is fussy and has a fever; his axillary temperature is 99.9ºF (37.7ºC). He has been cranky since last night.

Disposition: The mother is advised to take the infant to be examined today at the ED (weekend call). A 2-month-old infant with fever and fussiness should be checked soon.

A fussy infant of this age without fever should also be checked. A true fever is a rectal temperature ≥100.4ºF (38.0ºC).

## CASE #553

TIME: 9:32AM

A five-week-old female infant

CC: Cough & a decreased appetite
The baby has a cough and is feeding less than usual. She has no fever and no vomiting. Disposition: The mother is advised to take the infant in to be checked at the clinic today. A young infant with a cough should be checked.

## CASE #554

SPRING                                                                                         TIME: 12:05PM

A four-month-old male infant

CC: Constipation
The infant is constipated. He is not having daily bowel movements and his stools are hard.
Disposition: The mother is advised to give the baby more water to drink, to offer him juices like diluted prune or pear juice, and to observe. The mother is advised to introduce the new juices or solid foods one at a time. She may dilute the juice with water (one ounce of juice to 2-3oz. of water). She may substitute oatmeal or barley cereal for rice cereal. Hydration and fibers help produce bowel movements.

## CASE #555

SPRING                                                                                         TIME: 2:02PM

A one-month-old female neonate

CC: Facial rash & flatulence
The baby has a facial rash and has been passing gas frequently; she is on Similac with Iron formula.
Disposition: Without seeing the rash, it is difficult to say if it is consistent with allergic dry skin, heat rash, or neonatal acne. However, given the gassiness together with the rash, the mother is advised that cow's milk based formula might cause allergies, facial

rash, and colic. She is advised to try a soy based formula, like Prosobee or Isomil formula and to observe. In some cases, infants with cow's milk allergy are also allergic to soy proteins. In these cases, there is a protein hydrolysate formula (Nutramigen or Alimentum) that should be tried. In this neonate, it is unclear that the formula is causing the symptoms. The mother should also try to burp the baby more and to avoid using soap on the infant's face as this may be drying. The baby may be checked in the clinic.

## Case #556

A one-week-old male neonate

CC: Constipation
The mother states that the baby has not had any bowel movements in 14 hours. He is otherwise fine and is currently sleeping.
Disposition: The mother is reassured and advised to observe the baby. The mother may offer the baby small amount of boiled, then cooled, water to drink. She is to make sure he is taking adequate formula or breastmilk. The mother can also massage the baby's belly, bicycle the baby's legs and gently take a rectal temperature to stimulate a bowel movement if the other measures do not help. If the baby is comfortable, not cranky, not vomiting, and has a soft stomach, then he may be observed at home.

## Case #557

A seven-month-old male infant

CC: Feeding problem & vomiting occasionally
The baby has been on breastmilk, formula, and solid foods. Today, he has been refusing the breastmilk, but has been taking the formula and baby food well. The mother states that the baby has been vomiting intermittently for the last 3 weeks.
Disposition: The mother is advised regarding feedings. The infant should be checked to see what is causing his vomiting. If his weight is fine and he has been gaining weight properly, then the vomiting might be due to overfeeding or inappropriate feeding. The mother is advised to have the infant checked in the clinic as soon as possible. The infant should have a complete physical examination, including a neurological exam and a fundoscopic examination of the eyes.

## Case #558

Time: 10:35PM

A ten-day-old female neonate

CC: Separation of extra digit (finger)

The baby has one extra digit on each hand which had been tied off at birth and the extra digits are both separating with some bleeding now. Her skin is peeling and she has slight bleeding on the separated sites of the fingers. There is no redness nor discharge. Disposition: The mother is advised to keep the skin clean and to use Bacitracin ointment on the separation sites three times per day until complete separation and resolution.

## Case #559

Spring

Time: 12:15AM

A three-month-old female infant

CC: Cough & vomiting after coughing

The infant has had a cough and she has been vomiting afterwards. She was seen a few days ago by her physician and the mother had been advised to use nasal saline drops. Disposition: The mother is advised to give the infant Pedialyte instead of formula temporarily. She may give it in smaller amounts and shorter intervals so the baby can better retain it after coughing, and she is to observe. Once the infant tolerates the Pedialyte, she may then offer her formula but she should continue giving her smaller amounts at shorter intervals. Smaller amounts of fluids in the stomach are better retained after the forceful coughs. The mother is advised to continue to use the Normal Saline drops to the nose and to use a humidifier in the room around the infant; hydration keeps the mucous membranes of the respiratory tract moist and helps to alleviate the cough. While she most likely has a viral infection, a 3-month-old infant may possibly have a chlamydial infection, Bordetella pertussis infection, or bacterial pneumonia and so these should be considered. If the cough persists or if the baby has a fever, then the infant should be reexamined.

## Case #560

Spring

Time: 3:00AM

A one-month-old female neonate

CC: Nasal congestion & a medication question

The baby has nasal congestion. The mother would like to know if she can use Normal Saline nose drops.

Disposition: The mother is advised to use the Normal Saline nose drops 1-2 drops into the nostrils, three times per day for 3-5 days and to observe. The baby may be checked if the cold lasts more than five days, or if she were to develop any fever or cough.

## Case #561

Spring                                                                                   Time: 6:00AM

A five-week-old male infant

CC: Stuffy nose & fussiness

The infant has been having a stuffy nose. He has no fever. He also has been cranky.

Disposition: His father is advised to use a humidifier in the room, use Normal Saline nose drops in his nostrils (one to two drops three to four times per day, for three to five days), and to observe.

If he were to develop a fever, cough or continued fussiness despite the advised measures, then he is to be checked today.

## Case #562

Spring                                                                                   Time: 5:35PM

A five-year-old male child

CC: Fever

The child has history of asthma and he has a fever today. His temperature is 101.0°F (38.3°C); his mother wants to know if he can have Tylenol for fever.

Disposition: The mother is advised to give him one and one-half teaspoons of Children's Tylenol (160mg per 5mL) every 4-6 hours as needed for fever. She may also offer him fluids (water, juice, soup, ginger ale) and observe him. If he is coughing or wheezing, then she is to start his asthma medicine (albuterol).

## Case #563

Summer                                                                                   Time: 2:28AM

A two-year-old female toddler

CC: Fever

The child has a fever; her temperature is 101.0°F (38.3°C). There are no other problems. Disposition: The mother is advised to give her Children's Tylenol (160mg/5mL, one teaspoon every 4-6 hours) for fever, offer fluids (water, juice, soup, ginger ale), and to observe. She may be examined if the fever persists or it gets to be ≥102.2°F (39.0°C).

## CASE #564

SUMMER                                                          TIME: 5:45PM

A five-year-old female child

CC: Seizure & ear infection

The child has a known seizure disorder and is on Zonegran, yet her seizures are not well controlled. This call comes from a hospital ED in a different county within the state. The physician assistant states that the child has had a seizure lasting about three minutes and that she also has signs of an ear infection.

Disposition: He is advised to make sure she has no signs of meningitis. She should be stable (continue to be seizure-free with a normal neurologic exam, and normal vital signs) and treated for her ear infection and is to be seen by her neurologist. The child missed her appointment in the clinic today.

Meningitis is associated with fever, headache, vomiting and may be associated with a stiff neck or opisthotonos (an extreme extension of the neck and body). A child with signs of meningitis should have a spinal tap done and to be treated with appropriate antibiotics intravenously.

## CASE #565

SUMMER                                                          TIME: 5:44PM

An eight-year-old female child

CC: Abdominal pain

The mother states that the child has been complaining of intermittent diffuse abdominal pains in the last month. However, today she has been complaining of localized pain in right lower abdomen for about 20 minutes. She denies any fever or vomiting.

Disposition: The mother is advised that if the child has pain exacerbated by movement (pain that gets worse when she walks or jumps up and down) or that is severe, then she should be checked at the ED tonight. Otherwise, if the pain is mild and not getting worse with movement, she may be checked tomorrow. Abdominal pains that get worse with movements like jumping, imply that there is an intra-abdominal organic (organ related) pathologic condition (obstruction, inflammation, tumor, torsion, etc.) and so these patients should be checked urgently.

## Case #566

Autumn                                                    Time: 10:43PM

A 15-month-old female toddler

CC: Burn, first degree
The mother states that the child has touched the hot iron with her hand lightly and has resultant redness of the skin. The toddler is crying. There is no blister formation.
Disposition: The mother is advised to use a cold compress on the redness, to apply Bacitracin, to give her Infants' Tylenol (80mg) and to observe. The mother also is advised to avoid leaving the hot iron and hot foods or drinks where the child may gain access. Child-proofing the home also includes removing access to electrical outlets, small objects, button batteries, coins, medications, laundry detergents, and household cleaning liquids.

## Case #567

Autumn                                                    Time: 6:00 PM

A three-year-old female child

CC: Medication question
The child had been seen at the walk-in clinic and medication was prescribed for the cough and cold. Amoxicillin was given. Her father was not sure about the dose of Amoxicillin.
Disposition: The father is advised that at this age it depends on the type and severity of the infection. Amoxicillin is given based on the child's weight, 45-90mg/kg/day and in two or three divided doses. She was given Amoxicillin 250mg/5mL. She may be given one teaspoon every eight hours for 10 days for streptococcal pharyngitis, for example. However, for an acute ear infection with associated fevers, the higher dosing of Amoxicillin (90mg/kg/day) is recommended (two teaspoons of the same formulation thrice daily).

# CASE #568

AUTUMN                                                          TIME: 6:10PM

A two-month-old male infant

CC: Frequent stooling after having received immunizations recently
The infant had his 2-month-old immunizations yesterday. Today, it appears that he has
had eight very small bowel movements. The infant is breastfed.
Disposition: The father is advised and reassured. However, the baby is to be observed.
The mother should continue breastfeeding.
Breastfed infants sometimes have several bowel movements per day, but these should
not be in large amounts nor watery.


# CASE #569

AUTUMN                                                          TIME: 6:55PM

A three-month-old male infant

CC: Fever & cold symptoms
The infant has a fever, cough and a runny nose. He vomited the formula twice today.
His bowel movements are normal.
Disposition: The mother is advised to give him Pedialyte instead of formula for 6-12
hours, and then, when that is tolerated, she is to resume formula. For the cold, she
is to use Normal Saline nose drops (one to two drops into the nostrils, three to four
times per day for three to five days) and to use a humidifier in the room. For the fever
(temperature≥100.4ºF [38.0ºC]), she is to give him 40mg of Infants' Tylenol and to
observe. If the fever is ≥102.2ºF (39.0ºC), or if he is ill-appearing, or if he cannot
tolerate the Pedialyte, then he should be checked at the ED tonight.


# CASE #570

AUTUMN                                                          TIME: 10:05PM

An eight-year-old male child

CC: Medications question
The mother states that the child is on Risperdal 1 mg and that he has a history of
asthma. He appears to have cold symptoms today. The mother would like to know if
he may take his albuterol for cough/wheezing. She also wants to know if she may give

him Motrin if he were to develop a fever.

Disposition: The mother is advised that he can use the albuterol MDI inhaler (via spacer, 2puffs every 4-6 hours) for cough and wheezing and that he may have Children's Motrin (100mg/5ml, two teaspoons every 6-8 hours) for fever.

Risperdal is indicated for the management of irritability associated with autistic disorders in children/adolescents (5-16 years of age). There is also an indication for use of Risperdal in the treatment of bipolar mania in adults and in children older than 10 years of age.

## CASE #571

AUTUMN                                                        TIME: 10:17PM

A one-month-old male neonate

CC: Question about soy formula

The mother states that the infant is breastfed and that he is also given supplemental formula. She tried Isomil formula and it appears that the infant tolerates it better than the cow's milk based Similac formula. The infant was born at full term.

Disposition: The mother is advised that she may use Isomil formula as a supplement if she does not have enough breastmilk.

It is acceptable to give full term neonates a soy protein formula instead of a cow's milk protein based formula. It is not however medically indicated to make this substitution except in case of galactosemia, milk-protein allergy, lactase deficiency, or when the parents prefer that the infant have a vegetarian diet.

## CASE #572

AUTUMN                                                        TIME: 11:15PM

A two-year-old male toddler

CC: Cold & wheezing

The mother states that the child has a cold and fever and that he has been wheezing. He currently is sleeping comfortably. He has no history of asthma in the past. The cold started today and the toddler's temperature is 100.0°F (37.7°C).

Disposition: The mother is advised that if the child is coughing a great deal and is wheezing from his chest, then he should be checked at the ED tonight. However, if the noisy breathing appears to be due to nasal congestion, then the mother is to use Normal Saline nose drops one to two drops into his nostrils three to four times per day for three to five days. Also, she is to use a humidifier in the room, give him one teaspoon of Children's Tylenol (160mg) every 4-6 hours for fevers, offer him fluids (juice, soup, ginger ale), and observe.

## CASE #573

AUTUMN                                                      TIME: 9:36AM

An eight-year-old female child

CC: Exacerbation of asthma
The child has a history of asthma and started wheezing now.
Disposition: The mother is advised to start the albuterol metered- dose-inhaler (MDI) via the spacer, and give her 2 puffs. If she is still coughing and wheezing despite this, she may repeat the albuterol in 20 minutes. If this makes the child better, she may then continue the albuterol every 4 hours for a few days. When the child is better (usually in 3-5 days) she may then give her 2 puffs every 6 hours and continue doing so until she has no cough at all (usually for another 5 days or so). She is to offer her more fluids (juice, soup, ginger ale), and observe. If she is in any distress (rapid breathing with flaring of alae nasi, retractions and using the abdominal muscles to breath) or the albuterol is not helping her wheezing, then she should be seen at the ED.

## CASE #574

AUTUMN                                                      TIME: 10:12AM

A one-year-old male infant

CC: Post immunization crying & cold symptoms
The child had his Flu shot today and he has a runny nose. He is also crying more and coughing.
Disposition: The mother is advised to give him Infants' Tylenol (80mg), to use Normal Saline nose drops (1-2 drops into the nostrils, 3-4 times per day for 3-5 days), and to observe. She may also use a humidifier around the child. The injectable Flu vaccine is an inactivated virus vaccine and is not a live virus vaccine and so has few side effects. It is possible that the symptoms are a minor side effect from the vaccine, but more likely, because of the season and activity of the most respiratory viruses in autumn, there is a possibility that the infant has been exposed to a virus that would cause a cold.

# Case #575

Time: 10:24AM

An 18-month-old male toddler

CC: Insomnia
The father states that the child does not sleep at night. The child has a history of seizure disorder and is on Zonegran 150mg twice per day.
Disposition: The father is advised to prevent the infant from taking long naps during the daytime, and to also talk to his neurologist regarding his sleep. Zonegran may cause trouble sleeping (insomnia) and so together with the neurologist, they may consider changing the medication.

# Case #576

Autumn                                                    Time: 11:27AM

A three-month-old female infant

CC: Nasal congestion
The infant has been having nasal congestion. She has no fever.
Disposition: The mother is advised to use Normal Saline nose drops (1-2 drops into the nostrils, 3-4 times per day for 3-5 days) and to offer her fluids (water, white grape juice, and formula or breastmilk). The mother is also advised to use a humidifier in the room and to observe. She is to have the infant checked if she develops any fever or if the cold is not getting better in 5 days.

# Case #577

Autumn                                                    Time: 1:10PM

A six-week-old male infant

CC: Cough
The infant has a chest cold and congestion for 2-3 days. He has already been seen at the hospital twice and the mother has been advised, but he continues with nasal congestion and a slight cough. He has neither vomiting nor fever and is feeding and voiding well.
Disposition: The Spanish-speaking mother is advised via interpreter to use a humidifier in the room, to use Normal Saline nose drops 1-2 drops into the baby's nostrils, 3-4

times per day for 3-5 days, and to observe. Upper respiratory infections (URI) usually last about five to seven days. If the infant looks sick, is not feeding well, coughs a great deal, or has any fever (rectal temperature ≥100.4°F [38.0°C]) then he is to be rechecked at the ED (weekend call).

A neonate with any amount of fever should be checked

## CASE #578

AUTUMN                                                                                   TIME: 1:15PM

A 14-month-old male infant

CC: Fever & crankiness

The infant has a cold and a fever. His mother states that the fever appears to be persistent with temperature at 101-102.0°F (38.3-38.8°C). He has also been fussy.

Disposition: The mother is advised that the child should be checked. Rhinovirus infections are the most frequent cause of the common cold, and the peak activity of the virus is in the autumn and spring. Other viruses that can cause respiratory symptoms include influenza viruses, adenoviruses (which circulate all through the year) and respiratory syncytial virus (RSV). The infant with persistent fevers and fussiness should be checked.

## CASE #579

AUTUMN                                                                                   TIME: 1:42PM

A two-month-old male infant

CC: Nasal congestion

The infant has had nasal congestion for two days. He has had no fever.

Disposition: The mother is advised to use Normal Saline nose drops (one to two drops into the nostrils, three to four times per day for three to five days), She is to use a humidifier in the room and is to observe. Given his young age, the infant is to be checked if he were to cough, vomit or develop any fever (rectal temperature ≥100.4°F [38.0°C]).

## CASE #580

AUTUMN                                                                                   TIME: 3:08PM

A two-year-old male toddler

CC: Fever & croupy cough

The toddler has a fever and croupy cough (a barky cough) that started today. He has no vomiting and he is not drooling.

Disposition: The mother is advised to give him Children's Motrin syrup (100mg/5mL, one teaspoon every 6-8 hours) for fever and to give him warm fluids to drink (warm water, soup, flat ginger ale). She is to produce warm steam around him via humidifier or hold him in steam in the bathroom with the hot water running in the shower for five to ten minutes. She is to make sure he is getting better. He may be checked if the condition persists despite these measures or if he has noisy breathing. The viruses mostly responsible for croup associated with fever are the parainfluenza viruses and they are more prevalent in autumn.

## Case #581

Autumn                                                          Time: 3:46PM

A Two-week-old female neonate

CC: Straining & constipation

The mother states that the baby is straining to have bowel movements. She has not had any bowel movement for 2 days, but she is otherwise fine. The bowel movement was normal 2 days ago.

Disposition: The mother is advised to offer the baby some boiled, then cooled, water to drink and to ensure that she is taking adequate amounts of formula or breastmilk. Straining at early infancy is very common and the mother is reassured. She is also advised to make sure the baby is not fussy, that her abdomen is soft, and that she has no vomiting.

## Case #582

Autumn                                                          Time: 6:45PM

A 15-month-old male toddler

CC: Wheezing

The toddler was seen at the ED and has received medicine via nebulizer. He is currently sleeping comfortably. She does not know whether she should wake him to give him the medication he is due for.

Disposition: The mother is advised continue to give his medicine (albuterol) via nebulizer every 4 hours, around the clock as instructed and to offer him fluids to drink and observe. The mother is also advised to keep his appointment for follow-up.

## CASE #583

AUTUMN                                                    TIME: 7:32PM

A ten-month-old male infant

CC: Head injury
The infant fell while trying to walk and hit his forehead on the floor. He cried immediately after he fell and had no loss of consciousness; he has a small bump on his forehead.
Disposition: The mother is advised to put an ice pack wrapped in a towel on his forehead and to observe him. If the child vomits, if she is worried about him, or if he has any problems then she is to take him to the ED to be checked.

## CASE #584

AUTUMN                                                    TIME: 9:30PM

A 23-month-old male toddler

CC: Post-circumcision
The toddler had a circumcision recently and the bandage has just fallen off. There are no signs of infection.
Disposition: The mother is advised to use some Vaseline or A&D ointment on the site of circumcision area and to observe.

## CASE #585

AUTUMN                                                    TIME: 11:17PM

A one-week-old female neonate

CC: Colic symptoms
The baby has colic symptoms, unexplained crying at times. She cries after feedings and is bringing her knees to her abdomen at times. She is also passing gas. She is mostly breastfed and given Similac Advance formula as a supplement. She is otherwise well, feeding well and voiding well. Her abdomen is soft and she has not been vomiting nor spitting up.

Disposition: The mother is advised regarding the prevention of colic in the breastfed baby. The mother should refrain from drinking too much cow's milk and should avoid eating gas producing foods (like onion, radishes, beans and cauliflower). She should also avoid overfeeding the baby. Given the timing of the symptoms (relation with feedings), the mother may also try reflux precautions like holding the baby upright for 20-30 minutes after feedings, creating an incline (nothing in the crib but a sheet under the head of the mattress to create an incline), burping more frequently, and giving shorter or smaller feedings but with more frequency (shorter intervals in between). If these measures do not seem to help, then the baby can be checked by the pediatrician.

## CASE #586

AUTUMN                                                                    TIME: 5:45PM

A four-year-old female child

CC: Fever
The child has a fever; her temperature is 104.0°F (40.0°C).
She was seen yesterday by her pediatrician and has been on amoxicillin since last night for an ear infection.
Disposition: The mother is advised to give her Children's Tylenol (160mg/5mL, 6 mL every 4-6 hours) or Children's Motrin (100 mg/5ml, 6 mL every 6-8 hours) for fever, to offer her more fluids (juice, soup, ginger ale), and to observe. If the symptoms persist after 2 days or so while being on antibiotics, she is to be rechecked.

## CASE #587

AUTUMN                                                                    TIME: 8:28PM

A four-year-old male child

CC: Sore throat & eye discharge
The child complains of a sore throat and he also has been having eye discharge. He may have a slight fever; his temperature was not taken; he has no vomiting and no other problems.
Disposition: The mother is advised to clean the eyes with sterile water (use warm, boiled then cooled water), give him a teaspoon of Children's Tylenol (160mg/5mL), and have him checked tomorrow morning. Some serotypes of adenoviruses cause pharyngo-conjunctivitis and these viruses are active throughout the year.

## CASE #588

AUTUMN                                                    TIME: 11:25PM

A five-year-old male child

CC: High fever

The child has a fever; his temperature is 103.0ºF (39.4ºC). Tylenol was given three hours ago. He has no other symptoms nor complaints. He has no vomiting and is eating well.

Disposition: The mother is advised to give him Children's Motrin (100mg/5mL, 2 teaspoons every 6-8 hours) for fever, offer him fluids (water, juice, soup, ginger ale), and to observe. The child is to be checked tomorrow morning.


## CASE #589

AUTUMN                                                    TIME: 1:31AM

A three-year-old male child

CC: High fever & cough

The child has a fever; his temperature is 103.3ºF (39.6ºC). He also has a cough and he vomited once when he was crying. His mother gave him Motrin and has been sponging him with tepid water. His temperature has decreased slightly.

Disposition: The mother is advised that the child should be checked given the high temperature, cough and vomiting.

If the temperature is now below102.2ºF (39.0ºC), and his cough is not distressing, then she may give him a dose of Children's Tylenol (160mg/5mL), 6 mL, offer him fluids to drink (water, juice, ginger ale) and take him to be checked when the clinic opens in a few hours. Tylenol may be repeated every 4-6 hours for fever.

The dose of ibuprofen (Children's Motrin) for high fever is 10mg/kg per dose and may be repeated every 6-8 hours for fever.


## CASE #590

AUTUMN                                                    TIME: 7:45AM

A seven-month-old male infant

CC: Cough & wheezing

The infant has been having a cough and wheezing for the first time; his mother is an asthmatic.

Disposition: The mother is advised to take the child to the walk-in clinic (urgent care clinic) today to be checked and to receive bronchiolitis/asthma treatment.

## CASE #591

WINTER                                                                TIME: 5:46PM

A seven-month-old female infant

CC: Vomiting

The infant has been vomiting, she has had no fever; she has had normal bowel movements today. There is no blood and no bile in the vomitus; she is urinating well.

Disposition: The mother is advised to start Pedialyte in small amounts, to make sure she can retain it, and to observe. If the vomiting persists and the child cannot tolerate the Pedialyte, then the infant is to be checked at the ED tonight. If she could keep the Pedialyte down, she may continue the Pedialyte for 6 to 12 hours then start the formula and observe.

## CASE #592

WINTER                                                                TIME: 6:30 PM

A six-week-old female infant

CC: Congestion & cough

The infant had two watery stools, once yesterday and once the day before yesterday. She has been congested for three days and she has a slight cough; she has not had any bowel movements today.

She does not have any fever; she is feeding well and urinating well.

Disposition: The mother is advised that if the baby has a cough, she is to be checked at the ED tonight given her young age. Otherwise if she has no cough, she may be seen tomorrow morning in clinic. For the nasal congestion, the mother can use Normal Saline nose drops one to two drops into the nostrils, three to four times per day, and use a humidifier in the room. The neonate with a cough should be checked in a timely manner.

## CASE #593

WINTER                                                                TIME: 7:44PM

A two-week-old male neonate

CC: Separation of the umbilical cord
The mother states that the baby's umbilical cord is partly separated and that it smells a little.
Disposition: The mother is advised to clean the umbilical cord and umbilical stump with alcohol (isopropyl rubbing alcohol, 70%) and is to observe. If the condition persists and there is truly a foul smell, then the baby is to be examined.


## CASE #594
WINTER                                          TIME: 8:53PM

A 21-month-old male toddler

CC: Head injury
The toddler hit his forehead against the wall when he was running.
He has a slight swelling on his forehead. He cried immediately. He had neither loss of consciousness nor any other problems.
Disposition: The mother is advised to put an ice pack wrapped in a towel onto the swelling 15 to 20 minutes every hour and to observe. If he usually sleeps around this time of the evening, then she may let him sleep, but she is to make sure he can wake up and respond to the stimulation appropriately. Also, she is to see that he has no vomiting. If he demonstrates any abnormal behavior s or repeated vomiting, then he should be checked immediately.


## CASE #595
WINTER                                          TIME: 1:30AM

An eight-year-old male child

CC: Waking up screaming & a possible headache
The child suddenly awoke a couple hours ago screaming and is complaining of a possible headache. His mother states this is the second time that this has happened.
The first time was 2 nights ago. He was seen at the ED then and Motrin was advised. Tonight, after the episode his mother gave him Tylenol about 90 minutes ago, but the child is still screaming.
Disposition: The mother cannot hear the advice because of the loud screaming. She will take him back to the ED now. If the child has a headache, he needs to be

examined and evaluated. However, it is possible that the child has night terrors, also known as sleep terrors. Sleep terrors are partial arousal parasomnias, defined as episodic nocturnal behavior. Sleep terrors come on suddenly and usually occur in the first few hours of sleep. The conditions mostly happen during the NREM (non-rapid eye movement) part of sleep (partial arousal parasomnias). Nightmares are more common than night terrors, and these happen during the latter part of the night, when REM (rapid eye movement) sleep is more prominent. However, a child complaining of a severe headache warrants a thorough work-up.

## CASE #596

WINTER                                                                    TIME: 8:37PM

A two-year-old male toddler

CC: Croup & a history of asthma
The toddler has croup, hoarseness and he has a history of asthma. He is on asthma medicine (albuterol MDI), which he has been using via the spacer. He has neither fever nor vomiting.
Disposition: The mother is advised to use a cool mist humidifier around the child and to continue using the asthma medicine, albuterol MDI via spacer 2 puffs every 4-6 hours, for his cough. She is to offer him warm fluids (water, soup, ginger ale), and to observe. If he is not getting better or if he is in any distress, he is to be seen at the ED.

## CASE #597

WINTER                                                                    TIME: 8:45PM

A five-year-old male child

CC: Toothache
The child has been having a toothache.
Disposition: The mother is advised to give him Children's Tylenol (160 mg/5mL, 2 teaspoons every 6-8 hours as needed for pain), to rinse his mouth with water, and to have him seen by the dentist tomorrow.

## CASE #598

WINTER                                                                    TIME: 10:00PM

A nine-month-old male infant

CC: Fever

The infant has been having a fever today; his temperature was 102.2°F (39.0°C) about four hours ago, Tylenol was given and his temperature currently is 101.9°F (38.8°C). He has neither vomiting nor cold symptoms. He has been urinating well and is taking his formula well.

Disposition: The mother is advised to give him 80mg of Infants' Tylenol every 4-6 hours for fever, offer him fluids (water, juice, and formula or breastmilk), and to observe. If the infant continues to have a fever, especially if the temperature is ≥102.2°F (39.0°C), then he should be checked in clinic tomorrow.

## CASE #599

WINTER                                                    TIME: 12:32AM

A four-year-old female child

CC: Eye discharge

The child has eye discharge that started today. She has had no other problems except for mild cold symptoms. When she awoke this morning, the eyes were stuck shut because of the discharge. The child is currently sleeping.

Disposition: The mother is advised to clean the eyes with sterile water and to take her in to be checked in the morning at the clinic.

An eye culture might be done and proper eye drops will be prescribed. Given the child's cold symptoms, in addition to having the eyes checked, the child's ears will also be checked. Often eye and ear infections occur concomitantly.

## CASE #600

WINTER                                                    TIME: 1:10AM

A two-year-old male toddler

CC: Eye discharge

The mother states that the child has eye discharge that started today. There is a large amount of discharge.

Disposition: The mother is advised to clean the eyes with sterile water and to observe. The mother is to take him to be checked in the morning when the clinic is open. Adenovirus infections cause conjunctivitis, but sometimes bacteria may be the culprit. Therefore, when there is heavy eye discharge, an eye culture and susceptibility test may be done and the child is to be treated with antibiotic eye drops. Also, in young children who might not complain of ear pain, the ears should also be examined to rule out a concomitant ear infection. In older children, some providers may prescribe antibiotic eye drops over the phone after taking a thorough history.

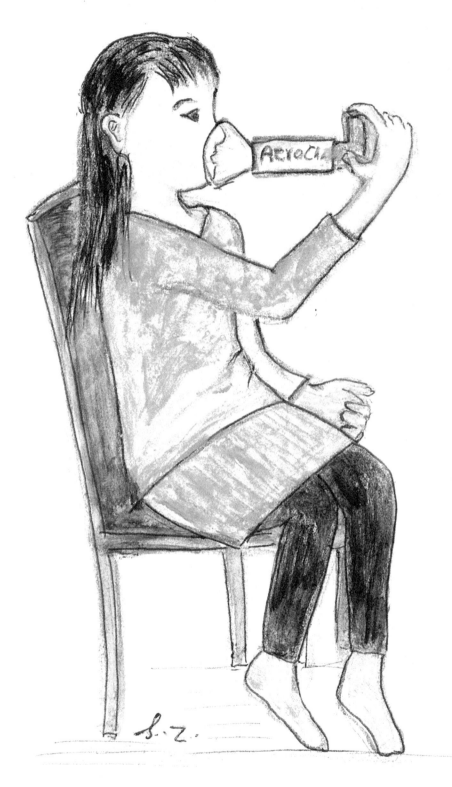

A child with Asthma

# Chapter Thirteen

## Case #601

A one-month-old female neonate

CC: Straining
The mother states that the baby has only one bowel movement every day and that she has been pushing to defecate.
Disposition: The mother is advised and reassured. Once daily bowel movements are normal if the bowel movements are of normal consistency and not too hard. Straining at the time of defecation in some young infants is common due to the lack of coordination between the increasing intra-abdominal pressures and the relaxation of the pelvic muscles, especially in neonates and infants below 6 months of age.

## Case #602

An eight-month-old male infant

CC: Diarrhea
The infant has been having diarrhea for a few days. His mother has been giving him Pedialyte and he is getting better. Enfamil formula has just been restarted and the infant had one greenish stool today.
Disposition: The mother is advised to give the infant Lactofree formula instead of Enfamil, observe him, and continue the Lactofree formula until he has normal stools

everyday. She can continue the Lactofree formula for two weeks. He may then resume the Enfamil. Due to some damage of the first layer of the intestinal wall during diarrhea; the production of lactase enzyme in those intestinal cells will not be sufficient after an episode of diarrhea, for this reason Lactose-free formula is preferred over cow's milk formulas after diarrhea. Lactose-free formulas and soy based formulas do not contain lactose; therefore, either of these formulas could be used.

## CASE #603

SPRING                                                                          TIME: 11:08PM

A five-month-old female infant

CC: Diarrhea & vomiting
The infant has been having diarrhea and vomiting since early this afternoon. She had one loose and watery stool and she has vomited twice. There is neither blood nor mucus in stool. She has had no blood nor bile in the vomitus; she has no fever and is urinating well.
Disposition: The mother is advised to start Pedialyte in small amounts and to offer it to her in short intervals (5-10mL every minute x 12 minutes). She may keep offering it to her in this fashion every hour. If she can retain the Pedialyte, then she may continue the Pedialyte instead of formula for 4 to 6 hours and then offer her Lactofree formula thereafter. She may also be checked tomorrow, in the clinic. If she can not keep the Pedialyte down, then she should be checked at the ED tonight.

## CASE #604

SPRING                                                                          TIME: 12:52AM

A five-year-old male child

CC: Fever
The mother states that the child has a fever; his temperature is 102.0°F (38.8°C). She is also asking for results from an MRI of the child's brain which was recently done for the second time.
Disposition: The mother is advised to give him Children's Tylenol (160mg/5mL, 2 teaspoons every 4-6 hours) or Children's Motrin (100mg/5mL, 2 teaspoons every 6-8 hours) for fever, to offer him fluids (water, juice, soup, ginger ale) to drink and to have him checked tomorrow. The MRI results, if available, will be discussed with her by the child's physician tomorrow.

# Case #605

Spring                                                                 Time: 4:46AM

A 15-month-old female toddler

CC: Fever
The mother states that the toddler has been having a high fever; her temperature was not taken. Tylenol has been given. However, she was given less than the dose required for her age and weight.
Disposition: The mother is advised regarding the correct dose of Infants'Tylenol (80mg every 4-6 hours) for fever. She is to take the temperature and give the Tylenol for temperatures ≥100.4ºF (38.0ºC). She is to offer her fluids (water, juice, flat ginger ale) and to observe the toddler. If the child continues to have a fever, then she is to be checked, especially if ≥102.2ºF (39.0ºC). The mother should use a rectal thermometer to take the temperature and should know that the rectal temperatures less than 100.4ºF (38.0ºC) are considered normal.

# Case #606

Spring                                                                 Time: 8:59AM

A 19-month-old male toddler

CC: Diarrhea & vomiting
The father states that the toddler has been having diarrhea and vomiting that just started today. He had one very loose stool and he also vomited once. There is no blood and no mucus in the stool; there is neither blood nor bile in the vomitus and he has been urinating well.
Disposition: The father is advised to start Pedialyte (in small amounts, sip by sip) and to make sure he can retain it. If the toddler cannot retain the Pedialyte, then he is to be checked today. If the vomiting stops, then the father is to continue the Pedialyte for 6 hours and then offer him foods like white rice, saltine crackers or graham crackers, applesauce, banana and plain yogurt. Fluids like Gatorade, white grape juice and ginger ale may also be given. He is not to offer him cow's milk for a few days. If he asks for milk, he may have Lactaid milk, and father should continue giving the Lactaid milk for one or two weeks. The toddler already has an appointment tomorrow in the clinic, which he may keep. If the child has blood in stool, is not voiding once every 8 hours, or has severe abdominal pains then he should not wait for that appointment and should be seen today.

A 13-month-old female infant

CC: Diarrhea with blood and mucus & fever

The infant has been having diarrhea and fever. The mother states that there is both mucus and streaks of blood in her stool. She has no vomiting. She is urinating well.

Disposition: The mother is advised to take the infant to the ED for stool culture and other lab tests. Pedialyte is advised as well as a bland diet for diarrhea (white rice, applesauce, banana and plain yogurt). The child may be given soy milk instead of cow's milk for a few weeks. For the fever, she may be given 80mg of Infants' Tylenol every 4-6 hours. Bacterial infections, anal fissures and an allergy to cow's milk are some of the causes of having mucus or streaks of blood in stool.

Soy protein based milk may be substituted for the cow's milk in the event of a cow's milk protein allergy. However, sometimes children are also allergic to the soy protein. Most diarrhea in children are due to viral infections. Diarrhea will cause a temporary lactase deficiency, and so cow's milk should be avoided (to avoid the milk sugars). A soy milk or lactose-free milk may be used.

Because this child has a fever associated with diarrhea and streaks of blood and mucus in stool, it is better to have her checked and obtain a laboratory work-up including a stool culture, and stool testing for ova and parasite. Among the pathogens that can cause diarrhea is Escherichia coli with at least 5 strains (Shiga toxin producing, enteropathogenic, enterotoxigenic, enteroinvasive and enteroaggregative). Shiga toxin producing E. coli (STEC) O157:H7 infections initially cause nonbloody diarrhea then bloody diarrhea after 3-4 days, as well as severe abdominal pains, hemorrhagic colitis and hemolytic-uremic syndrome (HUS).

Other pathogens are Shigella Species which are gram negative bacilli that cause diarrhea with minimal to severe constitutional symptoms (high fevers) and with associated mucoid stools, with or without blood.

Amebiasis is another intestinal tract infection that is associated with blood and mucus in the stool; the responsible pathogen is a parasite, Entamoeba histolytica, and is excreted as a cyst or as trophozoites into the stools of those afflicted. After the diagnosis is made, specific treatment will be given.

A child this age with blood in the stool should also be examined to see that there are no severe episodes of abdominal pains, as that may be suggestive of an intestinal intussusception. This may be diagnosed by ultrasound in the ED. This is when part of the intestine may telescope into another part of the intestines, which is very painful. If intussusception does not resolve spontaneously, then it may be treated by air contrast enema in the radiology department. If the intussusception is not resolved via air contrast enema, then surgical correction may be needed.

## Case #608
Spring                                                                    Time: 1:17PM

A two-year-old female toddler

CC: Diarrhea & vomiting
The toddler has been having diarrhea and vomiting since last night.
The mother did not respond to the return of her phone call, perhaps because the child was taken to the ED. Sometimes patients call just to inform the primary care physicians that the child will be going to the ED without necessarily seeking advice.
Rotavirus infection is associated with diarrhea and vomiting and it is more prevalent in toddlers and children attending daycare. It was much more common when the vaccine was not available. Currently there are two vaccines licensed and available which protect against Rotavirus. These are given orally at 2, 4, 6 months of age or just given at 2 and 4 months depending on which type of vaccine is available. The maximum age for receiving a Rotavirus vaccine is at 8 months of age, provided that is not the first vaccine in the series. The maximum age for starting the series is at 14 weeks and 6 days.

## Case #609
Spring                                                                    Time: 2:40PM

A three-year-old male child

CC: Streptococcal pharyngitis & azithromycin intolerance
The child is on azithromycin 200mg daily and has vomiting and a stomachache after taking the medicine. He has had strep throat previously and has been treated with oral penicillin for ten days in the past. Now he has developed another episode of streptococcal pharyngitis.
Disposition: The mother is advised that if the child cannot tolerate the medicine then he is to be reevaluated and may receive a penicillin injection. The mother also is advised to change the child's toothbrush after the 3-5 days of oral treatment. Also, the child should avoid sharing cups and utensils.

## Case #610

Spring                                                           Time: 3:44PM

A five-month-old female infant

CC: Infrequent stooling
The mother states that the infant has infrequent stool after her formula was changed to Neosure. She has been having two bowel movements daily; she wants to know if it is acceptable.
Disposition: The mother is reassured. Neosure is an enriched formula with increased protein, vitamins, and minerals compared to term infant formula.


## Case #611

Spring                                                           Time: 3:54PM

A 13-month-old female infant

CC: Blood & mucus in stool
The infant has blood and mucus in her stool. She has neither fever nor vomiting.
Disposition: The mother is advised to have the child examined and to have stool tests for culture and for ova and parasite detection, and perhaps some blood tests. The presence of blood and mucus in stool warrants having a physical examination and stool studies. Also, the possibility of a cow's milk allergy should be considered. Please see Case #607 for more information regarding infants and toddler with blood and mucus in stool.


## Case #612

Spring                                                           Time: 5:28PM

A 30-month-old female toddler

CC: Diarrhea & vomiting
The toddler has diarrhea and vomiting since last night. She has not had any fever; there is neither blood nor mucus in her stool. There is no bile and no blood in the vomitus. She urinates well.
Disposition: The mother is advised to offer her Pedialyte and clear fluids (Gatorade, ginger ale) and to observe her. If she cannot retain the Pedialyte, then she is to be seen at the ED. If the vomiting stops, she can continue giving Pedialyte and clear fluids and

give her foods like white rice, applesauce, banana and plain yogurt. The mother is to avoid offering her milk for a few days.

## Case #613

Time: 7:11AM

An eleven-week-old male infant

CC: Vomiting
The mother states that the infant has been vomiting after every feeding since about last week. The infant has had no fever and no diarrhea. There is neither blood nor bile in the vomitus. He is urinating well.
Disposition: The mother is advised to try Pedialyte. If he can retain it, she may then try Prosobee formula and observe. If the infant vomits after each feeding despite these changes, then he should be checked today. Emesis after each feeding could be the initial symptom of pyloric stenosis, the thickening of the stomach muscle which creates a blockage after the stomach, not allowing the food to pass. This entity can be diagnosed via ultrasound and requires surgical correction. The vomiting is nonbilious; it may be projectile and is progressive, occurring after each feeding. Males are more commonly affected than females. The vomiting associated with pyloric stenosis may occur as early as one week of age and as late as five months of age.

## Case #614

Spring                                    Time: 8:56PM

A three-month-old male infant

CC: Vomiting
The mother states that the infant has spit up all his formula today. There is no blood and no bile in vomitus. He has neither diarrhea nor fever. He is urinating well.
Disposition: The mother is advised to stop the formula and start clear fluids like Pedialyte. She is to offer him Pedialyte in small amounts and short intervals, and to observe. If the baby cannot retain the Pedialyte, then he is to be checked at the ED.

## Case #615

Spring                                    Time: 9:16PM

A six-year-old male child

CC: High fever & inhaled chimney soot

The child has a high fever; his temperature is 103.2F (39.5C). He has also been having a cough and some congestion. He had inhaled chimney soot two or three days ago.

Disposition: The mother is advised to give him Children's Tylenol (160mg/5mL, 2 teaspoons every 4-6 hours) or Children's Motrin (100mg/5mL, 2 teaspoons every 6-8 hours) for fever, to offer him fluids (water, juice, soup, ginger ale) to drink, and to observe. If he coughs a great deal or if the fever persists and is ≥102.2°F (39.0°C), then the child is to be seen at the ED, as an evaluation of his lungs is warranted.

## Case #616

Spring                                                           Time: 10:15PM

A two-year-old female toddler

CC: Cold symptoms including a cough & fever

The child has been having a cold, cough, and a fever since yesterday. Her mother gave her Motrin for fever and her temperature is coming down. She has had no vomiting.

Disposition: The mother is advised to offer her fluids (water, juice, soup, ginger ale) and Children's Motrin (100mg/5mL, one teaspoon every 6-8 hours) or Children's Tylenol (160mg/5mL, one teaspoon every 4-6 hours) for fever. Also, the mother is advised to use Normal Saline nose drops one to two drops into her nostrils, three to four times per day for three to five days. She should also use a humidifier in the room, and observe. The toddler may be checked if the temperature is ≥102.2°F (39.0°C) or if the cold is not getting better in five to seven days.

## Case #617

Spring                                                           Time: 2:55AM

A two-year-old male toddler

CC: Vomiting

The child has been vomiting for the past twenty minutes. There is no blood and no bile in the vomitus. He has neither fever nor diarrhea.

Disposition: The mother is asked if there is a possibility of any foreign body ingestion. She is asked if there is any associated fever or any other problems. If so, or if the vomiting persists, then he is to be seen at the ED. If not, the mother can try small amounts of water or Pedialyte and observe.

## Case #618

Time: 4:00PM

A 39-day-old male neonate

CC: Cough

The infant has had a cough for two days. He has had no fever.

Disposition: The parents are advised that if the infant has a cough, then he is to be examined. The neonate with a cough should be checked in a timely manner.

## Case #619

Late spring Time: 4:36PM

A six-week-old male infant

CC: Diaper rash

The baby has a diaper rash and the mother has noticed some blood on the skin around his penis. There are no other problems.

Disposition: His father is advised to clean the skin in that area and to see if there is a skin abrasion that has caused a spot of blood or if the blood is related to the retraction of the prepuce. Either way, he may apply Desitin or Bacitracin ointment to the area three times a day and have the baby checked at the clinic.

## Case #620

Spring Time: 6:18PM

A one-month-old male neonate

CC: Facial rash

The baby has had a facial rash on his cheeks for one week. He was born at full term. He is breastfed and given supplemental formula.

Disposition: The mother is advised not to use soap on the baby's face. If the rash is dry, she may use some Aquaphor ointment to the cheeks. If the lesions look like pimples, he may have neonatal acne for which no treatment is needed as it will self-resolve. Also, but less likely, the facial rash could be a reaction to the cow's milk protein in the formula.

The mother is advised to try a soy protein formula like Prosobee formula instead of cow's milk formula. Also, the mother can try to avoid drinking too much cow's milk and observe. The baby may be checked in the morning at the clinic.

## Case #621

SPRING                                                    TIME: 11:42PM

An 18-month-old male toddler

CC: Lump on the immunization site
There is a small painless lump at the site of his immunizations. There is no redness.
Disposition: The mother is advised to put a warm compress on the lump for about 15 to 20 minutes a few times per day as it will help to increase the blood circulation by causing vasodilatation and so will enhance the absorption of the immunization materials. It may take up to a couple of months for the lump to resolve and it may be a normal side effect from vaccinations.

## Case #622

SPRING                                                    TIME: 1:43AM

A two-week-old male neonate

CC: Crying at night
The father states that the baby cries a great deal at night. Currently, he is not crying. His bowel movements are normal and his abdomen is soft. His feedings are normal and he has been voiding normally.
Disposition: The father is advised regarding swaddling, cuddling and handling the baby. Sometimes infants may cry in the evenings, perhaps due to over stimulation. If there are no other problems, no fevers, normal feedings, and normal voiding, then the baby may be observed. If he cannot console the baby, however, then the baby may be checked.

## Case #623

SUMMER                                                    TIME: 8:30PM

A two-week-old female neonate

CC: Rash & a watery eye
The baby has been having a minute pimply rash around her neck. She also has one watery eye. She is otherwise well.

Disposition: The mother is advised regarding heat rash, and to avoid over warming the baby. Skin care advice is given. She is to bathe her and then pat dry her well. She may also put baby powder (not talc, but cornstarch powder) around her neck after placing some in her hand first (not directly to the area, to prevent inhalation). The watery eye could be a blocked tear duct. If there is eye discharge that is not watery, then the baby should be checked tomorrow.

Dacryostenosis is a condition in the neonates where the nasolacrimal duct is not completely open. Tears do not drain from the affected eye and so overflow, causing a watery eye. If there is no sign of infection (no thick discharge, no redness, no lash mattering), nasolacrimal massage two to three times per day helps to open the nasolacrimal duct. If the problem persists after the first birthday, then the infant will be referred to an ophthalmologist (eye doctor) at that point.

## Case #624

Summer                                                                                   Time: 8:55AM

A ten-week-old male infant

CC: Question about room temperature
The mother is asking if she can keep the baby in a room with air condition on.
Disposition: The mother is told that the appropriate room temperature for a baby is 22-26°C (72-78°F). She is not to put the baby directly in front of the air condition or any draft.

## Case #625

Summer                                                                                   Time: 12:00AM

A two-year-old female toddler

CC: Sore on the tongue & a slight fever
The child has been having a small solitary sore on her tongue and she may have a slight fever.
Disposition: The mother is advised regarding the diet. She is to offer her mild, soft foods and liquids, rinse her mouth with water after eating, and give her multivitamin drops (Poly-Vi-Sol) 1 mL daily.
The sore on the tongue could be because of a viral infection, due to irritation (from a hard or salty food for example potato chips), or may be due to a vitamin deficiency; therefore, palliative treatment (analgesia), avoiding further irritation of the tongue, and

the administration of a multivitamin will help. For the fever and pain, the mother may give her Children's Tylenol 160mg/5mL, one teaspoon every 4-6 hours. The toddler may be checked at the clinic later today.

## CASE #626

AUTUMN                                                          TIME: 10:00PM

A six-week-old female infant

CC: Nasal congestion
The infant has been having nasal congestion for one day, she has been taking the formula well, about 4-6 ounces every three hours. She has had no fever; her chest is clear according to her mother.
Disposition: The mother is advised to use Normal saline nose drops one to two drops into the nostrils, three times per day for three to five days, to use a humidifier in the room, and to observe. The neonate may be checked tomorrow if the mother so desires.

## CASE #627

AUTUMN                                                          TIME: 9:11PM

A four-month-old male infant

CC: Diarrhea
The infant has been having diarrhea that started today. He has no fever and no vomiting. There is neither blood nor mucus in stool. He is urinating well.
Disposition: The mother is advised to offer him Pedialyte for a few feedings instead of formula, then give him formula, and to observe.
If the infant continues having diarrhea, then he is to be checked. The mother may give him Lactose-free formula for one to two weeks.

## CASE #628

AUTUMN                                                          TIME: 12:39PM

A four-month-old male infant

CC: Question about the temperature of Pedialyte
The infant had been having diarrhea and her mother had called previously, Pedialyte

has been given and it appears that the infant is getting better. The mother has a question regarding the temperature of Pedialyte.

Disposition: The mother is advised to give the Pedialyte at room temperature; she may have the infant checked at the clinic.

## CASE #629

AUTUMN                                                      TIME: 1:25AM

A five-day-old male neonate

CC: Breastfeeding mother who is taking medicine

The baby is breastfed and the mother states that she had taken a Tylenol with codeine one tablet about 24 hours ago.

Disposition: The mother is advised to drink more water and use the breastmilk which was expressed before taking the medicine and to pump and discard the breastmilk for the next 24 hours. After 24 hours, she may breastfeed the infant. Codeine is a narcotic and causes drowsiness, respiratory depression and may even cause apnea. Thus, Tylenol with codeine is not recommended for nursing mothers.

Nursing mothers should always consult their physicians before taking any medicine, since many medications pass into the breastmilk and may cause adverse effects in breastfeeding infants.

## CASE #630

AUTUMN                                                      TIME: 6:58AM

A three-day-old male neonate

CC: Crying at times

The baby has been crying at times, mostly at night. He is feeding well, voiding normally and does not have a fever. His belly is soft and his bowel movements are normal.

Disposition: The mother is advised regarding appropriate feedings. If the baby is breastfed, then the mother should avoid drinking too much cow's milk and try not to eat gas producing foods like onions, radishes, cauliflower, and beans. She should have good feeding techniques and hold the baby in upright position for ten to twenty minutes after each of the feedings and let the baby burp and pass the gas from the stomach. She is to avoid overfeeding him and to help prevent him from swallowing air from the bottle or from prolong crying by swaddling, and gently rocking the baby. She may also create an incline in the bed by placing a sheet under the mattress at the head of the crib (nothing inside the crib). If these measures do not help, she may have the infant checked if she so desires.

## CASE #631

AUTUMN                                                                TIME: 11:30PM

A two-month-old male infant

CC: Constipation
The infant has been constipated for one week. He has no vomiting and no other problems. His abdomen is soft and he has been voiding normally. The last stool appeared to be normal.
Disposition: The mother is advised to give him some water to drink. She may also offer him one ounce of prune or pear juice diluted with water (2-3oz.) and observe. She may bicycle the baby's feet and gently massage the baby's abdomen in a clockwise fashion. To stimulate defecation, she may use the rectal thermometer with a small amount of Vaseline to take the temperature rectally. He may be examined at the clinic if the condition persists and a glycerin suppository might be prescribed at that time.

## CASE #632

AUTUMN                                                                 TIME: 6:00PM

A 30-month-old male toddler

CC: Nasal congestion
The child has a stuffy nose. He has neither fever nor any other problems.
Disposition: The mother is advised to use Normal Saline nose drops (one or two drops into his nostrils, three or four times per day for three to five days), to use a humidifier in the room at night, and to observe. He may be checked for fevers ≥102.2°F (39.0°C).

## CASE #633

AUTUMN                                                                 TIME: 7:26PM

A one-year-old female infant

CC: Fever
The infant has been having a fever; her temperature was102.0°F (38.8°C) three hours ago, Tylenol was given then and she currently has a temperature of 99.0°F (37.2°C).

She has no vomiting and no other problems.

Disposition: The mother is advised to give her fluids (water, juice, soup, flat ginger ale). She is to continue to give her Infants' Tylenol (80mg every 4-6 hours) or Children's Motrin (100mg/5mL), 100mg every 6-8 hours for fever. If the condition persists, or if fevers are ≥102.2°F (39.0°C), then the mother is to have the child checked.

## Case #634

Autumn                                                      Time: 10:16PM

A four-month-old female infant

CC: Fussiness

The infant has been cranky and has been pulling at her ears. She has no fever. She is breastfed and takes two and a half ounces of formula after breastfeeding. She has had no vomiting.

Disposition: The mother is advised not to overfeed the infant, to monitor her temperature, and to observe.

If the baby is fussy and is not consolable, then she is to be checked at the ED tonight. Otherwise, the mother may have her examined tomorrow morning in the clinic if required.

## Case #635

Autumn                                                      Time: 7:15AM

A seven-month-old male infant

CC: Question about the dose of antipyretics (medication for fever)

The infant has been having a fever. His temperature is 101.5°F (38.6°C). His mother would like to know how much Tylenol (acetaminophen) or Motrin (ibuprofen) she can give the infant.

Disposition: Tylenol and Motrin dosing is based on the age and weight of the children. Motrin may be given every 6-8 hours at a dose of 5-10mg/kg/dose. Tylenol may be given every 4-6 hours at a dose of 12-15mg/kg/dose. It is best to give the lowest dose that is effective. Generally, 10mg/kg of ibuprofen (Motrin) and 12 mg/kg of acetaminophen (Tylenol) are commonly used to calculate the dose as these are usually effective. A seven-month-old infant weighs about 13 pounds, or 6 kilograms. The mother is advised that she can give him 80mg (2.5mL) of Infants' Tylenol (160mg/5mL) every four to six hours for temperatures ≥100.4°F (38.0°C).

Alternatively, she can give him 60mg (3mL) of Children's Motrin (100mg/5mL) every 6-8 hours. Also, the mother is advised to offer him more fluids (water, juice, soup) whenever he has a fever. If his temperature is ≥102.2ºF (39.0ºC), then the child should be checked.

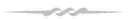

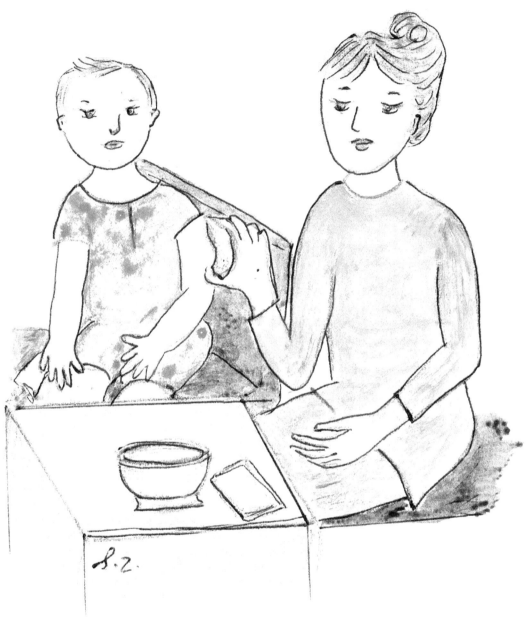

A child with a lump
on The site of immunization

# THE CHIEF COMPLAINTS
## ALPHABETICALLY

## A

Abdominal cramps
Case #328

Abdominal pain
Case #43, 72, 141, 181, 269, 470, 533, 565

Adolescent HPV
Case #499

Adolescent stomachache in an asthmatic
Case #279

Adolescent toe infection
Case #195

Adolescent pregnancy
Case #123

Adolescent question about the medication
Case #474

Adolescent vaginal problem
Case #133, 277

Allergies
        Case #52, 111, 162, 167, 210

Allergic reaction
        Case #480

Allergic rhinitis
        Case #391

Appetite (lack of, post infection)
        Case #214

Asthma
        Case #8, 10, 13, 14, 111, 135, 192, 201, 210, 219, 237, 296, 309, 355, 359, 365, 377, 389, 390, 395, 408, 411, 424, 466, 496, 573, 582, 590, 596

## B

Barking cough
        Case #330

Behavioral Problem
        Case #347

Bite (dog)
        Case #310

Bite (human bite, no broken skin)
        Case #31

Bite (insect)
        Case #37, 150, 174, 280, 527

Bleeding (prepuce retraction)
        Case #134, 519

Bleeding (following tympanostomy tube insertion)
        Case #129

Bleeding (vaginal)
        Case #133

Blood (in stool)
    Case #321, 607, 611

Bloody Diarrhea
    Case #403

Bloody Mucus in the diaper
    Case #65

Bloody Vomitus
    Case #49

Blister (toe)
    Case #160

Bump (back of the throat)
    Case #61

Burn
    Case #19, 489, 566

# C

Circumcision
    Case #584

Chickenpox
    Case #387, 419

Cold symptoms
    Case #5, 10, 20, 38, 75, 84, 96, 122, 124, 140, 171, 179, 191, 206, 218,
    220, 221, 229, 230, 231, 248, 267, 268, 285, 290, 292, 305, 308, 323, 368,
    382, 383, 386, 389, 390, 406, 421, 473, 482, 494, 498, 534, 536, 572, 578,
    616

Colic (neonate)
    Case #151

Conjunctivitis
    Case #9, 27, 89, 275, 399, 415, 433, 462, 503, 587, 599, 600

Constipation
    Case #50, 71, 117, 199, 242, 262, 374, 429, 434, 449, 464, 485, 554

Congestion
Case #147, 430, 576, 329, 349, 405

Congestion (nasal)
Case #529, 536, 579

Cough
Case #7, 24, 45, 53, 62, 69, 73, 81, 86, 106, 114, 122, 123, 130, 138, 145, 148, 164, 168, 187, 194, 204, 231, 232, 258, 267, 285, 324, 326, 336, 365, 368, 377, 380, 384, 386, 388, 395, 409, 411, 413, 416, 417, 424, 430, 440, 450, 463, 466, 496, 498, 510, 531, 559, 569, 615, 616

CP (cerebral palsy) with fever
Case #431

Cradle cap
Case #247

Crankiness (fussiness)
Case #6, 15, 23, 34, 85, 211, 245, 259, 471, 552, 634

Croup
Case #189, 330, 580, 596

Crying
Case #71, 125, 311, 458

## D

Dental decay
Case #238

Dental work
Case #436

Dental (loose tooth)
Case #542

Dental (toothache)
Case #597

Diarrhea
Case #15, 18, 20, 23, 33, 54, 66, 77, 79, 94, 95, 97, 100, 101, 155, 206,

223, 224, 227, 244, 246, 249, 255, 261, 265, 293, 298, 306, 313, 361, 385, 395, 410, 420, 426, 447, 476, 509, 535, 602, 603, 606, 607, 608, 612, 627

Diarrhea (post antibiotics)
Case #331

Dislocation of the shoulder
Case #63

Dizziness (adolescent)
Case #137

Dosage of the Antibiotics
Case #83

Dysuria (painful urination)
Case #139, 470

E

Earache
Case #2, 35, 39, 127, 225, 239, 325, 338, 352, 360, 392, 465

Ear discharge
Case #51

Ear drops substitute
Case #40

Ear drops intolerance
Case #113

Ear infection
Case #45, 46, 83, 158, 208, 222, 450

Eczema
Case #469

Enuresis (unwanted passing the urine)
Case #241

Epistaxis
Case #41, 208

Exposure to croup
    Case #550

Exposure to hepatitis (type unknown)
    Case #273

Exposure to strep throat
    Case #55

Excessive crying
    Case #278

Eye congestion
    Case #27, 275, 433, 503

Eye discharge
    Case #9, 89, 415, 462, 587, 599, 600

Eye foreign body (oil based perfume)
    Case #340

Eye (itchy)
    Case #30

Eye (pink)
    Case #105, 120, 338

Eye (swelling)
    Case #26, 193, 217, 250, 503


    F

Fainting (adolescent)
    Case #137

Feeding
    Case #88, 173, 207, 212, 276, 281, 364, 370, 557, 610

Fever
    Case #3, 4, 5 , 6, 7, 11, 13, 14, 16, 18, 21, 22, 25, 29, 36, 42, 47, 48, 51,
    55, 56 , 59 , 68 , 70 , 73 , 74 , 86 , 87 , 96 , 107, 114, 118, 121, 122, 123,
    132, 138, 146, 152, 155, 156, 158, 162, 163, 166, 168, 170, 175, 177,
    185,190, 198, 202, 204, 205, 211, 215, 223, 224, 225, 229, 230, 232, 233,

236, 246, 249, 252, 253, 256, 259, 263, 264, 265, 266, 268, 278, 289, 299, 302, 309, 337, 342, 343, 345, 346, 352, 353, 360, 365, 369, 372, 373, 375, 382, 383, 384, 388, 391, 392, 395, 396, 397, 402, 407, 409, 412, 413, 414, 418, 423, 431, 432, 439, 443, 444, 455, 456, 465, 466, 467, 468, 471, 495, 501, 502, 504, 505, 506, 516, 518, 530, 537, 540, 552, 562, 563, 569, 578, 580, 586, 588, 589, 598, 604, 605, 607, 615, 616, 633, 635

Foam in the mouth (neonate)
Case #44

Foreign body (skin)
Case #64

## G

Gagging the formula
Case #85

Gas
Case #92

Greenish mucus (nasal)
Case #56, 122

## H

Headache
Case #12, 28, 220, 302, 308, 391, 456, 540, 595

Hair loss (adolescent)
Case #404

Hematuria
Case #481

Hemoglobinopathy
Case #59

Hives
Case #52

Hoarse voice
Case #61, 546

How to give the medicine to a baby?
Case #78

How to take the temperature in an infant with diarrhea?
Case #80

Hydrocephalus with shunt (refuses to drink)
Case #183

# I

Ingestion
Case #49, 176, 256, 357, 401, 512

Injury (nail)
Case #371

Injury (eye)
Case #209

Immunization
Case #87, 112

# J

Jaw pain
Case #325

# K

# L

Laceration
Case #110, 538

Lack of an appetite
Case #334, 456, 534

Loose bowel movement (for two weeks)
    Case #435

Low oxygen saturation
    Case #60

Lump (in the neck)
    Case #81

## M

Medication (dose of Tylenol)
    Case #343

Medication (dose adjustment)
    Case #200

Medication (order)
    Case #180, 254, 314, 393, 394

Medication (question)
    Case #111, 245, 341, 342

Medication (refill)
    Case #282, 314, 356

Medication (side effect)
    Case #90

Mouth lesion
    Case #21, 93, 109

Mouth sore
    Case #128

Mucus (with cough)
    Case #164, 220

Mucus (in stool)
    Case #509

# N

Nausea
　　Case #337

Neonate (breastfeeding)
　　Case #207, 351, 491, 517, 549, 571

Neonate (cold symptoms)
　　Case #304, 442

Neonate (colic)
　　Case #151, 272, 283, 322, 472, 555, 585, 630

Neonate (congestion)
　　Case #147

Neonate (constipation)
　　Case #153, 295, 297, 312, 379, 400, 437, 441, 451,459, 513, 525, 539, 545, 556, 581, 601, 631

Neonate (cough)
　　Case #148, 194, 318, 376, 453, 553, 577, 618

Neonate (crankiness)
　　Case #295

Neonate (crying)
　　Case #58, 622

Neonate (diaper rash)
　　Case #619

Neonate (diarrhea)
　　Case #251

Neonate (excessive crying)
　　Case #363

Neonate (extra digit)
　　Case #551, 558

Neonate (facial rash)
     Case #115, 116, 151, 555, 620

Neonate (feeding)
     Case # 212, 438, 493

Neonate (fever)
     Case #22, 25, 152, 257, 332

Neonate (foam in the mouth)
     Case #44

Neonate (gas)
     Case #472

Neonate (greenish eye discharge)
     Case #548

Neonate (heat rash)
     Case #161

Neonate (lump)
     Case #483

Neonate (maternal HIV positive, on medication, extra dose of med. given)
     Case #234

Neonate (nasal congestion)
     Case #560

Neonate (rash)
     Case #363, 425, 460, 623

Neonate (runny nose)
     Case #547

Neonate (spit-up)
     Case #143, 363

Neonate (straining)
     Case #581

Neonate (stuffy nose)
     Case #561

Neonate (oral thrush)
        Case #165, 441

Neonate (umbilical)
        Case #188, 319, 335, 451, 593

Neonate (vomiting)
        Case #448, 522

Neonate (vomiting with underlying cleft palate)
        Case #159

## O

Ostensible pediatric call (mother calling for her own problem)
        Case #57

## P

Pain (leg)
        Case #372

Pain (right hip)
        Case #177

Pain (thigh)
        Case #32

Pain (tooth)
        Case #542

Pallor (pale skin)
        Case #343

Penicillin injection
        Case #18

Pharmacy Call
        Case #315, 398

Phlegm
        Case #323, 416

Pink Eye
Case #105

Pneumonia
Case #219

Post immunization
Case #87, 118, 157, 487

Post stomach virus gas
Case #92

Prescription (needed)
Case #99, 108

Prescription problem
Case #490

Pulling the ears
Case #16, 634

# Q

Question about the bowel movements
Case #524

Question about the bowel movements of neonate
Case #525

Question about dose of Tylenol (acetaminophen)
Case #170, 530, 605

Question about medication
Case #370, 446, 474, 500, 507, 526, 567

Question about the temperature of Pedialyte
Case #628

Question about prophylactic penicillin for sickle cell disease
Case #543

Question about the temperature of the room
Case #624

# R

Rapid pulse
    Case #60, 90

Rash
    Case #454, 488

Rash (allergic)
    Case #213, 354

Rash (Amoxicillin)
    Case #119, 508, 514

Rash (heat rash)
    Case #98, 126, 151,161,162,163, 167, 259

Rash (diaper)
    Case #270

Rash (facial)
    Case #115

Rash (facial and body)
    Case #271

Rash (fever and rash)
    Case #353, 373

Rash (round lesion)
    Case #300

Rash (following 3-4 days of high fever)
    Case #228, 506

Rash (one week after MMR immunization)
    Case #112

Refusing to drink
    Case #397

Respiratory problem
    Case #348

Roseola
        Case #228, 506

Runny nose
        Case #7, 73, 205, 272, 294, 329, 569

        S

Seborrhea
        Case #247

Seizure
        Case #502, 516 (febrile), 564

Sickle cell
        Case #324

Sinusitis
        Case #391

Skin infection
        Case #36, 107

Skin lesion
        Case #291, 301

Skin tag
        Case #445

Sleep problem (on Zonegran)
        Case #575

Sneezing
        Case #4

Soreness (corner of the lip)
        Case #169

Soreness (tip of penis)
        Case #178

Sore in the mouth
        Case #128

Sore throat
> Case #81, 138, 198, 263, 284, 423, 444, 587

Special needs child
> Case #452

Spit-up
> Case #417, 473, 614

Stomachache
> Case # 299, 302, 533, 609

Stomachache (adolescent)
> Case #279

Stomatitis
> Case #381, 492, 497, 514

Strain
> Case #461

Strep throat
> Case #486, 609

Stuffy nose
> Case #182, 198, 427, 505, 632

Swelling
> Case #8

Swelling (eye)
> Case #26

Swallowed a foreign body (sun flower seed)
> Case #49

## T

Teething
> Case #378

Thrush (neonate)
> Case #165, 216, 286, 441

Touching the ear
    Case #102, 196, 349

Trauma (finger)
    Case #344

Trauma (head)
    Case #1, 110, 316, 350, 457, 479, 528, 538, 583, 594

Trauma (nose)
    Case #477, 544

## U

Umbilical stump issues
    Case #149, 188, 319, 335, 451,593

## V

Vaginal (adolescent)
    Case #133, 142, 277

Vomiting
    Case #3, 12, 33, 51, 71, 76, 82, 87, 95, 97, 100, 101,103, 104, 131, 328,
    476, 484, 532, 533, 537, 541, 603, 606, 608, 612, 613, 617

## W

Wax coming out of ear
    Case #253

Wheezing
    Case #75, 187, 452, 531

## X

## Y

Yeast infection (vaginal)
    Case #142

Yeast infection (oral thrush)
Case #165, 216, 286, 441

Yellowish phlegm
Case #248

## Z

Zonegran (sleep problem)
Case #575

Zonegran (seizure disorder)
Case#564

# About the Author and the Illustrator:

Shahnaz Zomorrodian Erfani, MD, FAAP

| | |
|---|---|
| 1944 | She was born on October 25, in Tehran, Iran |
| 1960 | Won an Award 2nd place Prize in drawing and charcoal painting in Tehran |
| 1961 | Attended Painting Classes at Master Petgar's in Tehran |
| 1962 | Won an Award 1rst place Prize in drawing and charcoal painting in Tehran |
| 1963-1970 | Attended Tehran university, Medical School, became a Medical Doctor |
| 1969 | Married |
| 1971-1974 | Internship and Residency in Pediatrics, in New York City |
| 1976 | Passed the American Board of Pediatrics |
| 1977-present | Member of the American Academy of Pediatrics |
| 1976-2007 | Worked as a Pediatrician in the Bronx, NY. |
| 2007 | Attended Fine Art Class in Scarsdale, NY. |
| 1976-2010 | Lived in Scarsdale, NY |
| 2010-present | Living in California. |

# ABOUT THE EDITOR

The editor, Dr. Seamae Eghtedari Erfani is a practicing pediatrician, daughter of the author, and was born in New York City, NY. She was raised in Scarsdale, NY. She received her Bachelor's Degree and graduated with honors (cum laude) from Harvard University in 1996. She studied at St. George's Medical School and became a Medical Doctor, in 2000. She completed her Pediatric Residency at the University of Texas Medical Branch in Galveston, TX in 2004. She was an Assistant Professor of Pediatrics in the Section of Pediatric Emergency Medicine at the Baylor College of Medicine, in Houston, TX, from 2005-2008. Since moving to California in 2008 with her husband and children, she has been working at Kaiser Permanente where she helps children and their families thrive.

## Acknowledgements

I have many to thank. First and foremost, I must thank my beloved husband of nearly fifty years M. Hafez Erfani. Without his love, support and encouragement this book would not have been possible.

Next, I thank my family including my daughter Dr. Seamae Eghtedari Erfani for the countless hours she spent editing this book. Her husband, Dr. Mohammad Eghtedari, with his computer expertise, was also a great help. My son Dr. M. Sadi Erfani was also a tremendous help and a source of inspiration. My six grandchildren, Zachary Rumi, Hannah, Ryan, Isaac Arman, Ethan Rudaki, and Natalya Soraya are also inspirational for me. My lovely daughter-in-Law, Dr. Gail Salganick Erfani's support in the project was also a great gift. I love and thank them all for the comfort and joy they bring me everyday.

CPSIA information can be obtained
at www.ICGtesting.com
Printed in the USA
BVOW05*2035020218

506487BV00031B/192/P

9 781478 793816